I0435407

CONTENTS

Part 4: From 18-20 years old

Part 5: From 20-39 years old

Part 6: From 39 years old to present day

HEALING THE BROKEN PIECES OF MY LIFE

From *Broken* to Whole

France is a transformational author, speaker, Reiki healer and mentor.
She facilitates workshops with a mission to assist in
the uncovering and healing of the broken
pieces of your life.

Connect with her at

www.FranceBarringer.com

and claim your free one hour
Breakthrough session today!

FRANCE BARRINGER

ISBN: 1505826853
ISBN-13: 978-1505826852

PREFACE

As you are reading these words in this very moment, you may not consciously realize it, but your higher self has led you to these pages. You may call it your inner wisdom, intuition, spirit, guidance, or even providence. But the real beauty is that you have listened to the subtle whispers that have brought you here. You have acknowledged the "You" that on some level desires to be heard, understood, seen, and subsequently, healed and empowered.

In order to walk the path of growth, healing, and completeness with the past, we need someone we can trust to lead us through the present—because we can't do this alone. We need a teacher that can take our hand and be human with us.

The greatest of teachers do not say "follow me" but rather "I'll go first". Their courage to step into the unknown and hold a torch to illuminate our path is a gift beyond measure. Should you be so fortunate to meet such a teacher, you will have been one of the very few to have this privilege. Prepare to be one of the fortunate few.

France Barringer is much more than the author of this book. She is that once-in-a lifetime teacher that has walked the path and is now reaching out her hand, inviting you to take the journey that you have been reluctant to go on your entire life…until now.

Many authors write their life story, and as the reader, sometimes you feel like you are a detached, outside observer of their life. However, France's life story will awaken *your* story. The breadth, richness, and depth of France's emotions in her life are not unique to her—they are emotions that we *all* have felt on some level to varying degrees. Yet, so many of us have lacked the love, support, and compassion needed to unlock the vault of our inner most feelings that have been yearning to be noticed. But now, your imperfections are safe to emerge and come out in the open as France stands in hers with an honesty that is so refreshing and inspiring.

The true bravery of this book is the masterful way in which France shares her story with vulnerability and transparency that is to be admired. With organic and unfiltered emotions, France gets to the core of human emotion in a way that will grip you, push you to the edge, and evoke emotions rooted so deep within you that have been unconsciously running your life.

This book will uproot everything you have suppressed and ignored just to survive. France's story goes way beyond survival, and into the triumph of learning how to truly live by overcoming your biggest fears. This is an invitation for you to stop surviving, and start living life to the fullest.

It takes a wise soul to know that the thing that scares us the most is the thing that we're most meant to be doing. In this book, you will not only see how France faced her biggest fears head on by writing her story, but you will come to understand that her Divine purpose is to help you find yours.

And as you read France's story, you might think to yourself, "If France can overcome everything she did and find inner peace, it's time for me to look at myself and start living the life I was meant to live!"

As a testament to the authentic nature of this book, France asked me, her youngest son, to write this preface. As unconventional as this might be, it illustrates that time and again, she shows us the beauty of coloring outside the lines, challenging conformity, and how to find our own unique voice in a sea of humanity.

As you will discover, I have shared in much of my mom's journey. Yet, as I read her book, it felt as though I was hearing everything for the first time. With a purity and innocence that is so hard to find in today's world, I'm confident in saying that as you read this book, you will feel like you can relate to her. You will feel connected. You will feel emotions down to your bones. You will feel like you are not alone on your journey. You will feel a sense of hope, release, freedom, and excitement for what's ahead.

As her proud son, it has been a privilege to see my mom evolve into a teacher beyond my life, and that of humanity. And what I love most about this book is that France inspires in two ways.

1) By her example and how she's overcome adversity in ways that are nothing short of heroic.
2) By giving you very practical tools so that you can overcome *your* fears on the path to *your* healing.

Many times, people overcome great odds and leave us inspired, but do not share *how* we can do this in *our* lives. However, should you choose to transform your life, France has provided a guide book that will help you to face your biggest challenges and experience the healing, forgiveness, and ultimately, self love that waits for you on the other side. For once you can love yourself, love will flow to others in ways that are natural to the human spirit, not to the human mind.

I have often heard people say that it is a miracle that my mom turned out to be so vibrant and full of life given the challenges of her life. Yet, the real miracle is the one that lives inside each of us, ready to be awakened from its life-long slumber. This book will be your soul's alarm clock.

As a singer/songwriter, I have written many original songs. But there is one in particular that holds a special place in my heart called "Angel On The Ground" that I wrote for my mom. Once you read this book, you will experience how she can be an angel in *your* life. I believe Angels come in many forms. This one has come in the form of my mother.

Honoring you on your courageous journey,
Tiamo De Vettori

TESTIMONIALS

"As a Marriage and Family Therapist, I see the ongoing struggles of my clients when attempting to heal from past traumas/experiences and the effects on their current life situations and relationships. I too, like anyone else, am consistently searching for ways of healing my own traumas so I can assist others in healing theirs. Healing the Broken Pieces is a book I personally and professionally recommend to anyone who is struggling to heal their past in order to have a more peaceful present and successful future. France articulately, and vulnerably, shared her own life challenges and struggles and how she overcame them. France is one of those daring souls whose courage and openness is something only a select few would willingly create. The techniques and exercises in the healing guidebook were created to heal herself and all those she has come in contact with, including myself. France is not only a talented writer she is an experienced survivor, a wayshower, soul searcher and friend to all. If you are ready to take a leap in healing the broken pieces of your life, then you are ready to go on the journey of her life story and the steps she shares in her healing guidebook "Healing the Broken Pieces of my Life and Yours." I warn you, be prepared to cry, laugh, love and most of all HEAL."

Besan Hanna
Bilingual Arabic/English Marriage and Family Therapist

Spiritual Warrior, France Barringer, provokes with her two book series, "Healing the Broken Pieces of my Life" and her follow-up workbook, "Healing the Broken Pieces of my Life and Yours." Each is a masterpiece in its own right but together they are simply brilliant. A powerful tribute to life, and a spirit that cannot be broken, these books will most likely bring you to tears. Following France through her personal rabbit hole into spiritual maturation and the life that seemed to weave around her was heart-wrenching but true to form. She never failed to make me laugh, cry, and ponder with each riveting turn. This series is a rousing tribute to the pivotal role of choice and the importance of listening to one's heart. It is a must read for anyone who is serious about breaking the bonds that chain them and leaves in exchange the healing emotions of wonder, joy, compassion and hope. France truly is a light in this world and her books are a testament to the transformation that can occur. They have the power to change your life!

Chelsa Michelsen, M.S., Intuitive Astrologer

INTRODUCTION

The purpose of *"Healing the Broken Pieces of My Life"* is to provide healing into your own life. I believe that the healing of your mind, body and soul begins by honoring your life story.

One day, while writing my life story, I felt stuck. In frustration, I got up to take a break, and accidentally knocked a vase over onto the floor. It shattered into pieces.

As I sat on the floor picking up the broken pieces, *at that moment*, I realized that's how I felt inside, *broken and in pieces*.

I knew that, unless I was willing to look at each wounded part of me, and be pro-active in my healing, I might never feel whole and complete.

So, I picked up a pen and labeled each broken piece corresponding to the unhealed emotion that was still part of me. I named each piece one by one: Guilt, anger, resentment, fear, shame, bitterness and more until I uncovered all of the broken pieces inside of me. As I continued the writing of my life story, chapter after chapter, I honored each broken piece as part of who I was. As I did, unexpectedly, I was healing. I was transforming mind, body and soul.

I realized the reasons why I unconsciously created patterns of fear throughout my entire life. It started when I was 2 years old when the physical and emotional abuse began.

Two years ago, I almost died as I ended up in the ER with a heart beating three times faster than normal. I knew I had to make a change but I did not know how. Until…I started writing my life story.

The more I wrote, the more I understood the purpose of my sacred journey. I was finally honoring it. There was a healing power in recognizing and allowing the broken pieces to speak through me as I was writing about them.

Do you have broken pieces inside of you that might need healing? If so, I invite you to read about my own broken pieces first. You might recognize yourself in some of them. Together, we can uncover the healing power hiding behind the repressed emotions you may have felt your entire life. In darkness, all is hidden. In light, all is seen. Don't be afraid. You are not taking this journey alone, I am right here with you. Take my hand, and let's explore your broken pieces.

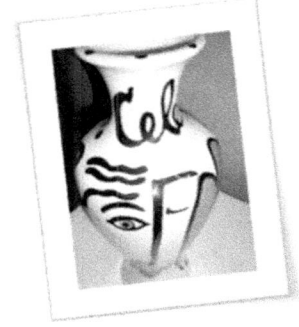

The other day, I bought myself a brand

new vase. It is also a reminder of who I am and who you can become: A new you, whole, vibrant, empowered, and unbroken.

The vase has a big huge red heart in the middle. It represents my mended heart rejoicing in the idea that I healed it and so can you. There is also an eye drawn on it, meaning that *I see you* and I know how you feel. I can show you the way, like I found mine. The word **Celebrate!** is written on the vase in big, bold, black letters which represents the celebration of the new you, the empowered being that you can become by following a step-by-step process that you can easily follow. That process has been developed into a healing guide, a companion of this book titled: *Healing the Broken Pieces of my Life and Yours.*

Sometimes, I open the box that contains my broken pieces as a reminder of who I was. They will always be a part of me. Yes, life is challenging at times, and if I revert to the pain I used to feel, I now know that I can create a better life without the unresolved emotions in my heart.

You don't have to live with the broken pieces in your heart. Like me, you can choose to live a transformed life. Are you ready?

Your task is not to seek for love, but merely to seek and find all the barriers within yourself that you have built against it. A Course in Miracles

Connect with France at:
www.FranceBarringer.com
Check the exciting free offers and **claim your gifts today**!

PART 1

FROM 2 TO 6 YEARS OLD

MY FIRST MEMORY - BROKEN PIECE: FEAR

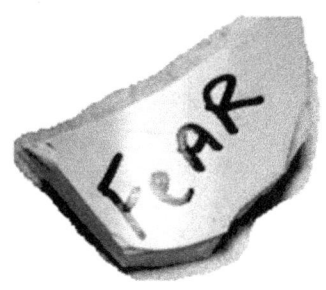

Lying in a crib asleep, I was awakened by my father who turned on the light hanging from the ceiling above me. As I opened my eyes, it was hard to see at first, as the light was so bright, but then, I recognized my father and mother standing beside the crib. My father was wearing a very dark long coat and a hat. My mother was covered in a brown fur coat and a matching hat. My father was hastily agitating me to wake up. I sensed anger in my father's eyes and simultaneously, I could feel my body hurting. In a gesture of power, he raised his hand and repeatedly hit my little body. I was hurting, and very afraid. I looked at my mother for comfort, but she remained unmoved.

And...that is the beginning of my journey. A journey that started a month before our winter officially begins in November. I was born in a small town in south-central Quebec, Canada. My father was a self-trained chef. Raised in a farmland, he was removed from school at a very young age to help his father cultivate the land. His education consisted of a sixth grade academic level, which is the equivalent to a first year level in Junior High School in the United States. He was five years younger than my mother.

My mother was his opposite. She was an educated nurse, only 4 foot 11" in stature, and weighed 90 pounds. She had short brown hair and hazel eyes. She was thirty-two years old when she married my father. I was the youngest of three daughters. I had blonde curly hair and blue eyes. My oldest sister Regine, who is three and a half years older than me, has brown hair and brown eyes like my father. Yvanne, the middle daughter, had straight light brown hair and blue eyes like mine. She was a year older than me.

After experiencing such intense emotions journaling my first childhood memory, I knew that in order to heal myself and my life, I had to continue this process no matter how painful it was going to be. I wanted to find answers to many situations in my life that I subconsciously kept re-creating. I had almost died two years prior, and there was no turning back. I wanted to live! Armed with determination and courage, I wrote my second memory in my journal.

MY SISTER

Being the youngest, I had to be in bed earlier than the others. One evening, there was a lot of commotion coming from the hallway. I could hear my sister's cries. I got out of bed and as I was standing in a nightgown at the end of the hallway, I saw my father sitting in a chair in the middle of the hallway and he was holding a bat in his hands. My sister, Yvanne, was at the opposite end of the hallway coming towards me, crawling on her hands and knees like an animal. As she was passing in front of him, he raised the bat in the air and hit her with it. She screamed out in pain, but knew to keep on crawling until he was done. And as she continued shuffling herself down that long hallway, he repeated the same gesture with the bat and hit her again. Yvanne told me later in life that our mother was hiding in the bathroom. When Yvanne would go and cry for help, my mother would rub her knees with rubbing alcohol and send her back for more.

I remember pleading for my father to stop. And that is the last I recall from that night. I was three years old and Yvanne was four. As we grew up, I was told by my oldest sister Regine, that Yvanne couldn't walk for as long as a week after these types of beatings, which occurred quite often. These were the so-called *disciplinary measures* used by our parents in the 1940's.

As I write about this second memory of my childhood, I now experience the fear all over again—along with anger, helplessness, and confusion.

My father bought a restaurant and kept it for two years before he went bankrupt. My parents had to pay a huge amount of money for my sister Regine, who was hit by a drunk driver while crossing the street when she was six years old. Very expensive hospital's bills forced my parents to declare bankruptcy. They were overwhelmed with debts to pay.

ABANDONMENT

Because of their financial difficulties, my parents left us in the care of two of my father's siblings. Regine and Yvanne were taken care of by my father's sister and my Uncle Camille, who had only one son, my cousin Jocelyn. Uncle Jules, my father's brother and his wife, Aunt Agathe, became my temporary guardians for one year. They

Abandonment

had two daughters, my cousins Sylvie and Luce. Not knowing them, at first I felt extremely sad, lonely, and I isolated myself. I invented a confidant out of a huge beautiful tree standing besides the house. It became my best friend. That tree was pure love to me, always listening.

I eventually adjusted to my new family and I have fond memories of the sweet smell of chocolate being stirred on the stove before being poured into a pie shell. The taste of that delicious, warm chocolate filled pie with a glass of cold milk was heaven to me. The sound of the harmonica played by Uncle Jules brought joy into my heart. I loved to play with my cousin Sylvie who is/was one year younger than me. My aunt was a very caring person and I remember her warmth, especially when she would comb my curly hair. I would see my sisters from time to time, but didn't see either of my parents for that entire year. My mother had found work in another city and my father was trying to find work elsewhere.

After one year of living with our relatives, the agreement between them and my parents came to an end, and they decided to place us elsewhere. The three of us were taken to an orphanage in Quebec City about 120 miles from the village where we were staying. My mother was renting a room at the mental hospital where she had found work. Once a week on Thursdays, we would spend the afternoon with her. Then sometimes on Sundays, she would visit us in the parlor of the orphanage where visitors were allowed.

The orphanage became our permanent residence for two years.

LIFE IN THE ORPHANAGE
5 YEARS OLD
BROKEN PIECE: NEGLECT

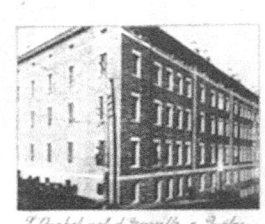

L'Orphelinat d'Youville à Québec

This new transition into a sterile, cold and unloving environment was very difficult. I felt abruptly cut off from everything and everyone Discipline was prevalent over warmth or affection. It was a very common and accepted practice to hit us on the hands and knuckles at any sign of possible disobedience. Yvanne and I were placed in the same group with other children around the same age. Being older, Regine was assigned to another group. It was forbidden to speak to one another and if by chance we crossed paths, we could only look at each other. I remember Regine crying each time she would see us. Sometimes, when I knew she was outside, I would run to the window to get a glimpse of her in the courtyard. I wanted to go play with her and I couldn't understand why it was not allowed.

Mealtime was a part of the day that I particularly disliked. At breakfast, we were forced to eat a disgusting, gooey, clumpy, bowl of slop. I had to restrain the urge of vomiting. I was not allowed to speak or leave the table until we were all done with the food. One of the nuns was standing by, holding a ruler, ready to hit any of us not eating the *gourmet* meal of the day. Sometimes, the memory of the smell and taste of the chocolate pie from my aunt and uncle's home would come back to mind. "Will that pleasure be gone forever?" I wondered, looking down at the gooey stuff I was forcing down my throat and regurgitating.

We wore uniforms and ugly brown heavy shoes that ripped the skin off the back of my heels, since the socks we wore had holes in them. Although my mother bought clothing for us, the sisters kept them from us.

I suspect that the lack of pretty clothes and shoes to wear was what ignited my love for fashion and style later on in life.

WHERE IS SANTA CLAUS?
BROKEN PIECE: TRUST

I had never heard of Santa Claus until I met Juliette. Juliette was a nun's aid who had a very keen ability for telling stories. One of those stories was about Santa Claus and how he kept a very special list for the well behaved children. On Christmas Eve, instead of coming down the chimney with gifts (like the Santa you might be familiar with), *this* Santa would travel with his elves and pick up those on his list to go back with him to the North Pole. One day, Juliette announced the names of the chosen ones. Oh my God, I was one of them! I was on Santa's list!

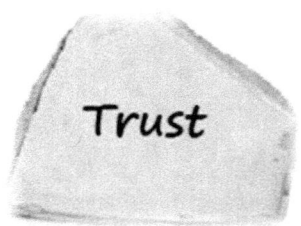

Filled with excitement, I could barely sleep at night. I visualized being on Santa's sleigh pulled by his reindeers and going way up in the sky with him. Can you recall when you felt such magical excitement in your childhood?

Daily, Juliette would remind us of the remaining days before Santa's arrival. The excitement leading up to Christmas Eve was almost unbearable. After months of anticipation, the day finally arrived. As I closed my eyes the night of Christmas Eve, there was no doubt in my mind that Santa was coming to take me with him. The next morning...

I woke up with the unexpected familiar sound of the bell ringing throughout the dormitory. As I opened my eyes, I shockingly realized that I was still in my bed and never left the orphanage. In disbelief, I looked around me and saw that the other kids were as confused and distressed as I was. Panic enveloped me. How could this be? Did we do something wrong? Why were we still here? Where was Santa? No one could answer these questions, but Juliette. Still in shock, I slowly started getting dressed for the usual day, crying my heart out.

We never found out what happened to Santa Claus, or Juliette. We never saw her again after that night. A few days later, a new sister's aid replaced her. I can't recall when I found out the truth about Santa, but I know that Juliette's lies had changed me forever. The naïve part and very nature of being a child had been taken away from me. But, I was also given a very powerful and valuable gift from that experience—*the ability to dream.*

When I became an adult, the capacity to stretch my imagination as I had done so many times with Santa Claus, led me to buy my dream home in the most unconventional ways. Without knowing how or when I could even buy a home, I accumulated beautiful, one of a kind pieces of furniture that fit perfectly into the new home I bought one year later.

My husband and I were living under a very strict budget at the time and the odds of qualifying for a loan were very slim. In fact, we were rejected the first time we applied for it. But in spite of the rejection, I maintained an unshakable faith that our loan would be approved. So, I wrote a letter to the underwriter explaining our unique situation and asked to be reconsidered. Two weeks later, I received a call from the lender telling me, "I have good news to tell you, we decided to approve your loan." Is an act of faith against all odds, the same as creating our own reality?

I manifested my dream home through the process of believing and creating it in my mind before it was even possible. It became reality to me and I did everything as though it was going to happen, no matter what. This was in 1992, many years before the movie "The Secret" came out into the world.

Regardless of how difficult your situation is today, look into the gifts that it can bring you and don't be afraid to use them. I promise you, it can change your life. *It changed mine.*

There is nothing like a dream to create a future. Victor Hugo

BECOMING THE QUEEN

After the crushing Santa Claus episode, I decided to rely only on myself to make things happen. A new goal of mine was to be crowned queen.

The nuns had just started a reward system. Each time a good behavior was noted, a hole was punched on a small card given to each of us. At the end of the month, the number of holes would be added up from each individual card, and the one having the most holes would be elected and crowned queen.

The crown, made of brilliant metallic green cardboard, was displayed on a desk in the classroom and was very much desired. Not only did I want the crown, but I also wanted the status of being a queen. But, there was a huge obstacle for that to happen. We were leaving the orphanage soon after the end of the month. I felt super excited about leaving, but I also knew that I only had *one chance* of becoming a queen. I remember thinking that, since the other girls were staying in the orphanage until they were 18 years old, they would have plenty of chances available to them. I had only a month left.

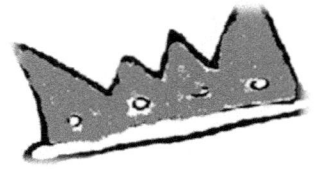

Racing against time, my card was only halfway filled with punched holes. But an idea came flirting in my mind one day when I realized that the hole punching device became defective. The regular circular holes were becoming less exact, and more and more jagged. Prior to this observation, I had broken a front tooth and it became very sharp and pointed. So, I practiced piercing holes on a piece of paper and noticed that the holes almost looked the same as the ones on the card! That's all I needed. If necessary, I would use my tooth to fill up my punch card. As the end of the month neared, such action became necessary. So, I filled up the rest of my card with holes given birth from my tooth and nervously presented it the next day to the Mother Superior. And to my elation and delight, I became the queen! That day in class, I got to wear my beautiful green, shiny crown for the entire day and yes, I felt like a queen. I was proud of my new elevated status from *orphan to queen!*

"The first one dressed in the morning," announced a nun one day "will be given a bag of candies." "Candies! I'll make that happen as well," I thought to myself. So at bedtime, I went to sleep with my clothes on and pulled the covers all the way up to my neck. The next morning, the bell rang as usual to wake us up, and while everyone was rushing to get dressed,

I simply got out of bed, ready to present myself to the nun with the candies. And of course, I got them.

From my perspective of the world, at seven years old, I was learning survival skills and building the determination to make things happen for myself. I realize now that the ways to achieve my goals were not completely pure, but how did I know the difference then? I couldn't count on Santa Claus, that's for sure.

Can you remember when you felt you had to survive on your own without counting on anyone but yourself? What did you do? How old were you?

PART 2

FROM 7 TO 13 YEARS OLD

MOVING IN THE MIDDLE OF NOWHERE

Two years had gone by since I was in the orphanage. My father found work in a small village called Franquelin, on the Northern coast of Quebec, Canada. It was only accessible by boat on the Saint Lawrence River or by helicopter. Here is a description of Franquelin taken from Wikipedia: 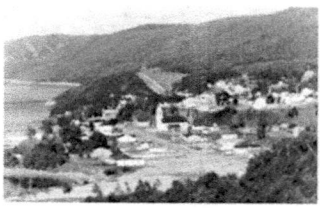 "Franquelin is a municipality in Quebec, Canada, in the region of Côte-Nord in RCM Manicouagan. Its population is 350 people over 530 square kilometers. Franquelin was founded at the foot of the Massifs rocks of the Laurentians where impressive cliffs plunge to the Gulf of Saint Lawrence.

Franquelin originated in 1911 thanks to the forest industry. The lumber would be transported to the rivers by horses. From there, it was shipped to paper mills in Ontario, and then later to Baie-Comeau starting in 1937. The Ontario Paper Company, owned by Colonel Robert R. McCormick, which later became the Quebec North Shore Paper Co., needed paper to supply the Chicago Tribune and the New York Daily News, which were also owned by McCormick.

Until 1961, when the road finally opened up to the closest town, the wood would be carried out onto a conveyer filled with water, and it would float to the wharf or quay, which was then loaded onto a pulp boat. From there, the wood would be shipped to the paper mills.

My father was hired by the Quebec North Shore Paper Co. He was in charge of cooking for the lumberjacks who lived in the camps.

Franquelin, being surrounded by forest, was infested with millions of mosquitoes. Every summer, the villagers had to cover themselves from head to toe to prevent being eaten alive by the blood sucking black flies. Your face had to be covered completely, except for 2 small holes for the eyes and a small hole for the mouth.

One day in September of 1955, my parents having saved enough money, released us from the orphanage. From the city of Quebec, we took a boat and navigated all day and all night to finally arrive at Franquelin, the village where I was going to live for the next ten years. I was seven years old at the time. From the quay, I could see a man wearing a white cap and apron. It was my father that I hadn't seen in years. I was happy to be free from the orphanage, and being with my mother and sisters created a sense of unity and belonging. We had finally arrived at our destination and our new residence; a halfway burned house that my father was in the process of reconstructing. I fell asleep that first night, with the sound of the rain falling into buckets located throughout the house. My mother's screams of terror awaked me. A mouse had crossed over her body. We all hastily got up and helped my father put traps all over the house in order to catch the uninvited guests.

Little by little, from his own hands, my father rebuilt a house that had burned three times in the past. Not only did it become habitable, but it evolved into a pretty white and blue house, perched on a hill with a beautiful view of the St-Lawrence River. There were beautiful trees outside and green grass in the backyard. We even had a blue and white swing that my father had built beside a small pond.

My mother, being a nurse, became the doctor of our village. She opened up an office in a small area of the house where she offered free consultations for patients and administered the necessary care. She ordered medications and medical supplies through vendors who came to the village or placed orders via phone or mail. We had one telephone line that we had to share with twelve of our neighbors. We had a specific ring assigned to each family to identify who the call was designated for. If it rang twice, it was ours to pick up. In the meantime, the other eleven families could listen to our conversations if they wanted to—all they had to do was lift the hand receiver and listen in.

We had two schools in the village--one for first grade through junior high and the second for high school. There was no sufficient heating system in the school I was in, so we had to keep our coats, hats, and mittens on indoors during the ferocious winters. There was no bus to pick us up either, so we really had to bundle up to walk two miles a day to go to school.

Very often, I watched my mother leave in a snowstorm when she was called on an emergency. The roads were blocked sometimes for days after a snowstorm. I often felt a sense of pride about her willingness to help others in need. Although I was not inspired to become a nurse myself, I had to help when an emergency presented itself. Such was the case one day when a lumberjack had accidentally cut his finger with a saw while cutting a tree. When he arrived at our home, he was being supported by two other men and the blood was gushing out of his hand. The poor man was in a lot of pain. He was so pale, weak, and ready to pass out. They had already made a long trip coming down from the forest. My mother actually saved his life since he would have bled to death. She asked me to stay with her to help. Nervously and as fast as I could, I gathered what was needed from her office: peroxide, gauze, tray of emergency tools, tourniquet, and morphine. I knew the routine. But this time, at nine years old, I was being apprenticed as my mother's assistant in a very big way. The blood had to be stopped immediately. As I rushed back, I saw that the lumberjack was about to faint. My mother told me, "France, hold this end of the tourniquet" while she twisted the other end in a knot to stop the blood flow. The finger was cut in half. She sterilized the wound, bandaged it, and injected him with the pain medicine while I was calling the emergency hospital at the closest town twenty-five miles away to send a helicopter over. My mother, in a moment of brilliance, froze the half-finger that was cut and sent it in a container with the patient to the hospital. The surgeon was able to sew his finger back. Later, an article was written in the town newspaper about my mother. It said something like this: "A remarkable nurse from the village of Franquelin saved a man's life today. Not only did she save his life, but his finger that was cut in half." That's what I admired most about my mother—her courageous acts in dramatic situations.

Although my mother had established herself in the village, she always remained very secretive and to herself. She didn't relate to people in the village and felt very isolated. I often saw her cry when she would reminisce about being in Quebec and how she longed to be back in the city that she loved so much. For forty-five years, she felt isolated the entire period she lived in Franquelin. I often felt like her; isolated and depressed.

Unlike her though, I enjoyed making new friends, and one of them came in the presence of a pretty grey cat that arrived at our door one day. I fed it and it kept coming back. We adopted her and named her Grisou, which is a French name that was a testament to her grey fur. I loved my cat very much.

Grisou had total freedom to come and go as she pleased in the village, and one day she got pregnant. In the basement of our home, there was an opening through the cement on one side of the wall. In that opening, I built a bed for Grisou so she could be comfortable giving birth and have a safe place to keep her newborn kitties. I made sure she had a fresh bowl of milk beside her bed. Grisou knew about that special place since I took her there many times to get her familiar with it. One day as I was looking for her, I found her lying down in that place, breathing differently. It was time for her to give birth. I stayed with her until her babies were born. I was excited to be part of such a magical event. Grisou gave birth to four beautiful little kitties.

FORCED TO KILL
BROKEN PIECES: GUILT, SHAME

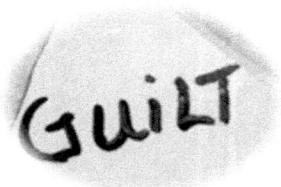

A week after the birth of the kittens, my father came home from the camps. Unfortunately, he went downstairs in the basement and found the kitties. He was infuriated and told Yvanne and I to get rid of them immediately or he was going to kill them. He told us, "Either you do it, or I'll do it." And then he said, "If they are still here when I come home tonight, I'll get rid of the other one too" (meaning Grisou.) We had to make that happen and fast. Yvanne and I started going around asking our friends, our neighbors, and anyone we could think of that might want to adopt the kitties. No one was interested.

We didn't know what to do, so in desperation, we sought the advice of an older friend, Diane. Surely, we thought she would be wiser and could help us find a solution. As time was rapidly running out, we ran to her home to consult with her. She was thirteen years old, Yvanne was ten, and I was nine. "What choice do you have?" Diane asked us. "No one wants to adopt them. You can't leave them outside or they will die. If your dad comes home and sees them, for sure he will kill all of them. So this is what I think is best. We have to get rid of the kitties ourselves, but not make them suffer. Let's put them in a potato bag and drown them. But before we drown them, so that they won't suffer, I will bang them against the rocks and that will kill them immediately. They are so little, they won't feel a thing." "No, we can't do that! That is horrible," I said. Then Yvanne said, "Well, you know what is going to happen if we don't, so, we need to do it ourselves. We have to be tough."

We continued talking and since we couldn't find a better solution, we concluded that it was the best of two evils. At least we would save Grisou's life. Anxiously, we all went home to get the kitties. We packed their little bodies in the white cotton potato bag and the three of us left for the beach. When we got there, Diane chose a huge standing rock and asked us to help her. Yvanne and I told her we couldn't go through with it. I felt so nauseous and wanted to vomit. Holding the bag, Diane desperately started banging the kitties against the rock. The most horrific scene unfolded in front of my eyes. The kitties were crying, and when I saw the potato bag turning red, I closed my eyes. I covered my ears with both hands, but I could still hear them. Those were horrible, never-ending moments. Why were they not dying? It was not supposed to happen that way! Diane screamed, "They are not dying! We need to drown them!" and she finished them off that way. I don't remember what we did with the bodies. I don't remember even walking home that day. All I knew was that we had become murderers! That day changed me forever.

At dinnertime, my father came home and told me to go clean up the mess I had left in the basement, which was the little bed, the blanket, and the bowl of milk. Grisou was not there. With the life sucked out of me, I put everything in the trash can outside and went to bed crying myself to sleep.

The next day, I confessed to Grisou what I had done. I held her in my arms and asked her to forgive me. I think that she did, since she was still affectionate with me. Affection that, of course, I felt was undeserved. And even though Grisou seemed to forgive me, the tremendous guilt I felt could not allow me to forgive myself.

The irony of it all is that approximately one month after that tragic day, Grisou didn't come back home. I never knew what happened to her, and I ended up losing her anyway.

Recently, I was having lunch with a loving, compassionate friend of mine. I was telling her about the book I was writing, and specifically the episode with Grisou. So many years had gone by since that day, and yet the pain was coming up all over again. My friend interrupted me and asked, "Which color was Grisou?" "Grey," I replied. "Look outside the window," she said. A beautiful grey cat was nonchalantly walking right by the window where we were sitting.

Coincidence? I don't think so. The Universe is always sending us messages in different ways. The message that came while I was looking at the cat spoke loudly and clearly. I believe it was Grisou's way of saying, "I have forgiven you. Now it's time for you to forgive yourself."

I often think of how easy it is to judge someone who does something wrong in our eyes. If anyone would have seen Diane, Yvanne, and I that day, one would have passed judgment on us as being very cruel and sadistic children that were inflicting pain upon animals. Were we cruel children? Or was cruelty done onto us? How could we have known the difference? *What is the real truth behind any act of cruelty?*

We often judge, condemn, and punish, but the root of the problem remains. Where do you stand in your own life? Are you quick at judging others, or are you open to looking

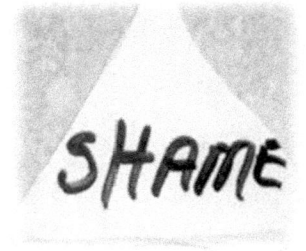

beyond what you see? And just to be clear, I am not saying that cruelty done to any human being or animal is acceptable. Absolutely not! However, just remember that when you judge another harshly, you may be in their shoes one day. Because of this and other reasons I have shared, I believe that, "Judgment against others weakens the truth about you."

During that period of time of my little life, I experienced deep feelings of depression and I was having horrible cramps in my stomach. I suffered from what we call today irritable bowel syndrome, and because of malnutrition, I had constant nose bleeds and cramps in my legs. I frequently had strep throat with high fevers. My neck was filled with swollen glands. Looking at Louise Hay's book, *Heal Your Body*, one can easily relate to the symptoms I was experiencing at the time. Nose bleeds connect with a need for recognition, feelings of being unrecognized, unnoticed, and crying out for love. Abdominal cramps signify fear as a probable cause. Cramps translate to tension and fear as well as gripping and holding on. A sore throat often means holding in angry words and feeling unable to express oneself.

Those symptoms and many others that I experienced throughout my life, indicate to me that they are all surrounding the same issues of fear, anger, anxiety, hopelessness, and not being able to express my feelings.

In my guidebook, *Healing the Broken Pieces of My Life and Yours*, I will help you to discover the relationship between your emotions and the physical ailments in your body and how to heal them.

ALL THAT GLITTERS IS NOT GOLD

It was Christmas Eve, one month after my 12th birthday. The tradition in the village was that on Christmas Eve, families gathered around the table to eat a light dinner and go to the midnight mass. After the service was over, families gathered together again, to eat a more elaborate meal... a sort of buffet, displaying different food selections. It was followed by the sharing and opening of gifts. Music and dance often ended in the early morning hours. This celebration was called the Réveillon.

I specifically recall that particular Christmas Eve, when I was twelve years old, because our neighbor had invited my sisters and I to go to their Réveillon. I was anxiously hoping that my father would allow us to go, since we didn't celebrate this festive custom in our home. For no particular reason, my father said no. Christmas for him meant winning the competition for the most beautifully decorated house in the village.

He had won the 1st prize for the past three years, since the beginning of the competition. Each year, the house on top of the hill, our house, was illuminated with beautiful shiny multicolor flashing lights and decorations. That Christmas Eve was no exception. My father had gone to the village's committee meeting and the votes were unanimous; he had won the first prize again.

My mother had prepared a very simple dinner, a Canadian meat pie to warm up in the oven and eat upon my father's arrival. Afterwards, we would all go to the early mass service at 6:00 pm. My father had told my mother when he had left early that day to not worry; he would be on time for dinner and take us to church.

Why my mother still believed in what my father said, is beyond me. Unkempt promises are the norm for an alcoholic. Of course, in 1960 the behavior of an addicted personality was not well documented or well understood.

My dad arrived around 8:00 pm that evening, in a drunken state, with the 1st prize award attached to his jacket. My mother looked at him with such disappointment in her eyes. He mumbled a few things and went straight to bed. My mother obviously was relieved that he was safe, but also very stressed out. She decided to go rest, as well, and left us to ourselves to warm up the pie and eat without them. Merry Christmas! Ho! Ho! Ho!

The main goal of Christmas had been accomplished! Ironically, the house on top of the hill was still proudly flashing its multicolored Christmas lights, while my sisters and I were trapped inside and felt its darkness.

19

The gloom of the night was even more emphasized, when I looked out our kitchen's halfway-frozen window and saw my neighbor's Christmas tree flashing through his living room window. I imagined the children opening up their carefully wrapped, colorful gifts. I heard imaginary laughter and could picture looks of surprise on their faces. I wondered how it would feel to be one of them. I turned around and looked at my sisters. Regine was playing a card game called Solitaire and Yvanne was listening to the radio. I didn't have to wonder how it felt to be one of us. Santa had bypassed us again that year.

How do you usually celebrate Christmas in your home? Is it important for you to be with your family and share the bonds of closeness and love? Are beautifully wrapped gifts your main focus or the love that your carry in your heart?

Remember that all that glitters is not gold. Can you see beyond someone's happy appearances on the outside? That person could be crying on the inside. Can you illuminate that person's heart?

PART 3

FROM 13 TO 17 YEARS OLD

NOT GUILTY, PUNISHED ANYWAY

As we became teenagers, my father's strict disciplinary measures continued. We were not allowed to be alone with boys and had to be supervised at all times. My oldest sister was the *chaperon* and she took her role very seriously. She was my father's favorite and my mother's right hand. My father added a beautiful bedroom in the basement for Regine. This made perfect sense since Regine was their oldest and favorite daughter. Favoritism was just one more way to control and manipulate our emotions. For example, my parents gave Regine gifts for her birthday and Yvanne and I, on rare occasions, got a $5 bill from my father, while he bought Regine a record player.

Not only did my father use Regine as a chaperon, but he also designated spies in the village that reported back to him about our activities. So, one of his favorite things to do when he came home from the forests was to go to the bar, have a beer with his friends, and hear all the gossip about us. Whether the gossip was true or untrue, it did not matter—my father believed his friends over anything we would say in our defense.

One of the false accusations made against us was that, while my parents were away for a day, Yvanne and I were apparently seen in the village with teenage boys and we took them home with us. That certainly infuriated my father.

When he came home that evening, he warned us of the impending punishment for our unforgivable behavior. We were doomed and we were going to get it good! He loved to create such dreadful anguish, anxiety, and fear in us. He even added more suspense by telling us, "It's going to happen before I leave, but you just won't know when." After two days of anxious waiting, he finally called on us. We had two girlfriends over that day for protection, thinking that maybe he wouldn't dare hurt us in front of them.

He, of course, out-thought us by sending them home. First, he called on Yvanne to come downstairs. Fearful, Yvanne asked, "France, can you go first?" "I might as well get it over with now," I replied getting up to go downstairs.

As if he were going to be merciful and believe me, my father asked me to tell him the truth about the boys. "Would it matter?" I dared to ask him. He immediately punched me in the mouth, splitting my lip open with the huge zodiac ring he was wearing. Blood was gushing out. He ordered me to go in the corner, stay on my knees, and not to cry or I would get hit some more if I did. Then, he called Yvanne to come downstairs. The sounds of my father beating her and her screams were intolerable to me. What torture! Finally, it was over. We went in the bathroom to wash our faces and my oldest sister and my mother were there. They told us, "You deserved it! Next time, maybe you'll listen."

A few minutes later, my father called on us again. As if he had some remorse for what he had just done, he offered us a $1.00 each to go buy candies at the local store. "I don't want anything from you," I told him defiantly. What else could he possibly do to me after this? Yvanne insisted that I take the money for her, and we both left for the store. Bruised and cut, we were going to buy our chocolate rewards. On the way, we encountered some friends of ours. "What happened to your face, France?" one of them asked. "I fell downstairs," I replied. Back then, abuse was a very common and accepted *well kept secret*. And in many cases, I'm sure it still is today. The exception being, it is now punishable by law. But when I was growing up, the parents *were* the law, especially in a very small village in the middle of nowhere.

This was the last time I remembered his physical cruelty. However, his psychological, sadistic ways of inflicting pain on us remained. On one occasion, my father kept us isolated for six months. We could only go outside to go to school or to church on Sundays. When you are thirteen years old and you can't go out and be with your friends, six months feels like an eternity.

On Sundays, we were forced to go to confession. To confess what? More of what we *didn't do* and then be punished for it? I remember confessing to the priest that I had said *maudit* (dammit), in English. For that, I had to say a rosary on my knees to be absolved from my sins so that I would not burn in hell for eternity.

How comforting! I thought. "After leaving this hell on Earth, you go into *another one*, except that hell is *even worse* since you remain there, burning for eternity." At a certain point, I had made up my mind. I couldn't listen to this nonsense about *God* anymore. I decided to find my own answers. And I did! I read many books on the subject outside of the fear-based religion I was born into. And I found a very loving and comforting God in the process. How about you? What is your God made of? Fear or Love?

Even when we were finally allowed to go outside, we lived in constant fear of being seen by one of my father's detectives, especially when we had boyfriends. Once, I was seen on the beach walking hand in hand with my fifteen year old boyfriend. My father's "spy" immediately reported back to him what he had seen and of course, when I got home that day, I knew I was going to be severely punished. As soon as I arrived, he confronted me with his usual anger and threats. For the first time in my life, I realized that I was no longer afraid of him. He slapped me in the face, and I spat on him declaring, "You will never hurt me again." He reacted by running to my mother, desperately untying his tie, asserting that he couldn't breathe and that he was having a heart attack. After that incident, I heard my parents one night discussing the possibility of sending me to a disciplinary home, since they couldn't handle me anymore. The fact that my mother agreed to that possibility deeply hurt me. "How could she not even fight for me?" I thought. But then again, she never stood up for herself, let alone for us, while my father was around anyway.

PLANNING MY ESCAPE

I decided I had to escape. In the summer of my 13th birthday, I packed my bag and was ready to leave home for good. I was planning on escaping from the small bedroom window that opened up to the roof of the house. From the roof, I was going to jump to the closest tree. I had it all planned, and I had practiced my jump to perfection. On a set day, I was going to meet with a male friend of mine at a local restaurant. Together, we were going to hitchhike to the closest small town. From there, my boyfriend's brother and his wife were going to pick me up and take care of me. I was determined to change my miserable life. That day for my escape came. As I was proceeding to escape through the window, Yvanne came upstairs and saw me. She begged me not to leave and went to get my mother to stop me. My mother was very upset and was crying, pleading for me to stay. I did stay-- mainly for my sister, I think. Still, the thought of leaving home was always present in my mind. As soon as I could, I did.

FROM ONE PRISON TO ANOTHER...

My first husband was a copy of my father. One may think that from the *lovely* memories I had of my father, I would try to stay away as much as possible from anyone that resembled him, but sadly, this would not be the case. I started dating his copycat when I was seventeen years old.

PART 4

FROM 18 TO 20 YEARS OLD

MY MARRIED LIFE

At the age of eighteen, I became engaged to my future husband. He was a bit taller than my father and a good-looking man. Not only did he possess some of my father's physical characteristics, but he was also an alcoholic and a very angry man, especially when he was drunk. He went into furies and scared everyone around him. Subconsciously, I was trying to get the love from him that my father never gave me. But, I was only repeating the violent patterns of abuse with a different person. When one is unaware, this is a common behavior in abusive relationships. This man was in love with me and I had value in his eyes. But I was "Looking for Love in All the Wrong Places" as the song goes. When I got pregnant the first year of my marriage, I became very afraid of his raging behavior. And when he was drunk, it was like he was possessed by demons.

One such episode that comes to mind is when I was eight months pregnant with my first son. We were on our way back home from a day spent at my in-law's house. He had been drinking all day with his buddies, while I was spending time with my mother-in-law. When he came to pick me up to go back home, I didn't realize how drunk he was. On our drive home that night, there was a snowstorm and I attributed his driving mishaps to the snow building up on the road. That is, until he opened his mouth.

I asked him not to drive so fast since I was afraid of the storm. But then, he became enraged and started screaming at me at the top of his lungs. I became very frightened. It was not safe for me to be with him in the car, or on the road, or at home for that matter. I felt trapped, again. I asked him to stop the car. Of course, he wouldn't. So, I opened the door, and when he slowed down immediately, I threw myself out onto the snow bank. Then, I walked back in the snow to his mother's house to get refuge.

After that night, I gave him an ultimatum; either you stop drinking, or I get a divorce. After that, he stopped for a few months, but then the nightmare started all over again.

GIVING BIRTH

On my eight and a half month pregnancy appointment, my doctor informed me that he would be leaving for vacation. He advised me that it would be best to induce the birth before he left. He ordered a procedure to be done in the hospital and gave me a prescription to accelerate the labor process.

And what did I know, but to follow my doctor's recommendation? I was pretty ignorant about the birth process back then and I had no idea what to expect. One must keep in mind, that forty-five years ago, living in the middle of nowhere, information was not readily available, as it is today. I was told that giving birth was going to be painful and that was the extent of what I knew.

So, while my husband was busy looking at cars that day, I walked from the doctor's office to the hospital. Upon my arrival, I was led into a room that looked like an operating room, with huge lights hanging from the ceiling. I got undressed, changed into a white hospital gown, and was told to lie down on the table under the big lights. I felt so cold. Being very afraid, I asked one of the nurses, "What are you going to do? My doctor didn't really explain anything except that a procedure to induce labor needed to be done." Showing me an instrument that looked like a long, sharp silver letter opener, she replied "We need to break the water and to do so, we need to insert this into your uterus." "You are not serious," I said in disbelief. "Isn't it dangerous?" "S'il-vous-plait madame, laissez-nous faire notre travail," she replied impatiently, which means "please madam, let us do our work," as if she had given me a very long dissertation on the subject. Unsure, I reluctantly lifted my legs in the air as I was told, and she proceeded to insert that scary object inside me. "A la grace de Dieu!" I exclaimed—an expression often used in French to attract the favors of the Divine when a perilous event is about to occur. Then I felt the cold piece of metal penetrating me and simultaneously, I felt some warm liquid coming out. When it was done, the nurse simply said, "Okay, get your prescription now and go home. In a few hours, when you feel enough pain, come back to the hospital."

I got up, put my coat back on, and walked to the pharmacy. It was the month of April, when you begin to feel Spring in the air, but it was still chilly that afternoon. As I was walking, I could still feel the water running down my legs. I walked faster on my way to the pharmacy and continued down the hill towards home. When I got home, I packed a small suitcase for two to three days and called my mother to tell her that I was going to have the baby that night. Then, I waited for my husband to come home. I had taken the pills to accelerate the labor and I was already in a lot of pain. When my husband finally arrived, he drove me to the hospital and left me at the doorsteps. Giving me a kiss goodbye, he nervously said, "I hope you understand, I am very afraid of hospitals." And off he went to his parent's home twenty miles away. I saw him again three days later when I was discharged to go home with the baby.

I checked myself in at the front desk. I was put in a room with another woman who was obviously in a lot of pain since she was screaming her head off. "Oh great," I thought, "something to look forward to when I'm giving birth!" The nurse gave me a white gown to change into and told me to lie down on the bed and wait.

Although I was afraid to know the answer to my question, I ventured to ask the woman who was in the room with me, "How long have you been here, my dear?" In reply, all I heard was a very loud scream. "All right, I got it. I'm sorry for what you're going through," I told her, fearing my own imminent pain. "Oh my God! Could I survive such agony?" I thought as I resigned myself to listening to her, while looking outside my window. It was very windy that evening and I was fortunate, because there was a tree by the window. Following its swaying movement comforted me. I didn't feel so alone.

Two hours had gone by when the nurse came to transfer the poor shouting woman to another room. "Thank God she is leaving," I thought. Soon enough, it was my turn to scream. The pain was increasingly getting worse. The nurse came back to check on how dilated I was. "You are at four centimeters," she said. "Oh horror!" I thought. Five hours had gone by and I was only at four centimeters? "Oh God help me!" I cried.

But, there was no help to be had. The nurse left again. By then, I was very afraid, in a lot of pain, and I felt so alone. For comfort, I looked outside for my tree, but it had disappeared in the darkness of the night. Around 10:00 pm, the nurse came back to roll me away in a wheelchair. I was moved closer to a small room adjacent to the delivery room. The room contained a bed and four bare, cold walls. I asked the nurse if I could keep my watch on as I felt that it was my only connection to the outside world. She obliged my request, closed the door behind her, and said, "We'll come back later to check on you." "Well, that's reassuring," I thought, feeling even more alone now without my window. The pain was so severe. I seriously thought I was going to die right there on the bed in that room and nobody would even know.

I found out later that taking medication to activate labor intensifies the pain. The hours were interminable. It was 2:00 am when the nurse came back to check the centimeters again. "Nope, it's not time yet," the nurse said. "So much for taking those damn pills" I cried. And one more time, she closed the door behind her without saying a word. Another hour went by and I couldn't wait for the door to open again. There was no button to push, no one could hear me, and I had to wait. Periodically, the nurse would come back: 3:00 am, 5:00 am—still not ready. At 6:00 am, she said, "It's getting there," and left again. At 7:00 am, she said, "I will call the doctor soon. It's getting closer." I was agonizing…and out of breath. Then around 8:00 am, finally, I heard some good news as the nurse announced, "It's time to move you into the other room now."

My ankles were strapped down by one nurse, while the other nurse was trying to reach the doctor. Then, I heard her say, "As soon as you see him, tell him that we are ready and to hurry up." The telephone was on a small table in the delivery room and I could hear everything the nurse was saying. That created more anxiety in me realizing that he was not even in the hospital yet. The nurses were pretty agitated and were calling other departments in the hospital to find him. Still, no doctor.

I thought, "Could it be that he had already left for his vacation and forgot all about me?" Then, I remembered what happened to Santa Claus in the orphanage. In the meantime, I was finally dilated at ten centimeters and ready to give birth…sixteen hours later. Determined to wait for the doctor, the nurses unstrapped my legs and crossed them over each other to stop the delivery process—not once, but three times. The third time, I pushed one of the nurses and ordered them both to not come close to me. This barbaric method of suppressing the birth of my baby had to stop. "No more waiting for the doc!" I screamed as the doctor finally arrived. And that's how my little baby boy was born.

"I am so sorry," he said, "got into traffic." At that point, I didn't care. Looking at my baby and hearing his cries for the first time was all that mattered to me. When I held him in my arms, the ordeal I had just gone through magically vanished. Oh my God, he was the most beautiful baby I had ever seen. He was absolutely perfect! His beautiful blue eyes even opened and were looking at mine. A connection between mother and son was forever established.

That day, I promised myself to give my son a better life than the one I had lived, up to this point. Keeping him away from an abusive environment was the first step. More than ever, I was determined to change my life. My mother had kept her three daughters in a very unsafe and abusive home because of the choices she made. For reasons unknown to me, other than her religious beliefs, my mother never divorced my father. Forty-eight years is a long time to live a miserable life! Regardless of my mother's circumstances, I am grateful for the precious gift that I was given—life.

When was the last time you thought of your life as being a miracle? A gift? Against millions of odds, you were the one that made it. You purposefully met your mother's egg and became the human being that you are today. Are you living your life with the same kind of determination and purpose?

Yes, life is very challenging at times. But just like giving birth is a painful and difficult process, by seeing the opportunity in the challenges you are facing, you will be born anew from each experience according to the perspective you choose to have today.

Surrendering to the process of birth throughout all its contractions and pain will free you from the "womb" that can no longer contain you. Every day you are given a new chance to outgrow what you once were. Give birth to yourself—the new you that wants to emerge and evolve. By no longer resisting the flow of life, you become a co-creator with the life force that moves you.

What are you waiting for? Do it today. How about right now? Give birth to that project you put aside. Quit that job you hate. Be brave and live your dream. Read that book that inspires you. Go on that vacation. Climb that mountain. Call your mother and say "Thank you." Yes, your mother. She is the one that ultimately gave you life. Thank your father too, you carry half of his DNA and without him, you wouldn't exist either. Live one day without judging yourself or others. Better yet, be brave and write your life story. You may remain anonymous after you write your masterpiece, if you choose to, but share it with the world! Make a difference in someone's life. I hope I will make a difference in yours.

I've had many broken pieces in my life and I have shared just a few of them with you, in this part of my story. I'm hoping that you'll follow along in the following segments of my life and join me in my healing journey.

Until then...
If you want to become whole, allow yourself to be broken.
If you follow one direction, allow yourself to be lost.
If you want knowledge, allow yourself to be ignorant.
If you want to shine, allow yourself to be a common stone.
Allow everything.
Resist nothing.
Create all things.
And when your work is done,
Take not the credit,
And it will last forever.

PART 5

FROM 20 TO 39 YEARS OLD

THE NIGHT THAT CHANGED THE COURSE OF MY LIFE

Two weeks after the birth of my son, I immediately went back to work. Paid maternity leave was not part of my benefits. My husband, being in a non-drinking phase, gave me hope of living a normal family life. That hope had taken months to build and suddenly, in one evening was ripped away from me.

My day started as usual. We had a family routine established. After work, I picked up my son at the babysitter, fixed the evening meal and waited for my husband to come home so that we could share the events of the day together, over dinner.

After feeding my one year old hungry little boy and realizing that my husband was running late, I started to eat my dinner. Many fearful thoughts came to mind as I mechanically put the food into my mouth. Unable to resist the dread that came over me, nauseated, I threw away the rest of my food. I looked at the clock. He was two hours late.

Many thoughts crossed my mind. Was he involved in an accident? Surely, someone would have called me by now...unless something was wrong with the phone. I picked up the phone and listened to the dial tone... it was normal. I quickly put it down, fearing that someone might call and would get a busy signal. 7:30 pm...and still no sign of him.

Around that time, I usually gave my son his nightly bath. He loved to play with his little toys floating on the water. One of his favorite things was trying to catch the soap bubbles that I blew up into the air. He burst into laughter when he saw them disappear into nothingness. We both would laugh and together, loved that nightly ritual. After I showered him with kisses, I put him to bed. He usually fell asleep after hearing his nightly lullaby that went like this: "Bonne nuit cher tresor, reve aux anges d'or....ending in ta maman sera la." Translating in English means: "Good night my treasure, dream of golden angels...and when you wake up in the morning, your mommy will be here." 10:00 pm. The front door opened. Moving towards my husband, I realized that my fears were founded. He had been drinking again. My stomach twisted in knots. I was familiar with the apprehension that I used to feel around my father. I saw the drunken evil-possessed eyes looking at me. "Where is my dinner?" he stormily blurted out, looking at the unset table. "I'm hungry." "It's in the fridge", I responded. "Just warm it up." "No! You are going to warm it up for me and you are going to serve it to me now!" he commanded, angrily pointing his finger at me.

I felt as though I was faced with an angry dog growling at me. Hiding my fear the best I could and without defiance in my voice, I replied, "I'm going to bed now. I need to go to work tomorrow." As I moved away towards the bedroom, he grabbed my arm and bullied me against the wall. He never physically abused me, but I knew the potential was there. He circled his hand around my neck, and as if a sudden dark idea flashed in his mind, he released me and walked towards my son's room yelling, "You are going to pay for this! I'll show you who the boss is around here! I'm taking my son with me and you'll never see him again."

"On my life!" I thought. Fearing for my son's safety, I ran to the kitchen and picked up the sharpest knife I could find in the drawer. I was ready to stop him no matter what I had to do. "If you take one more step, I swear, I will plant that knife in you" I screamed, holding the knife in front of his belly. "Give me my baby and get the hell out" I yelled, as I reached out with my free hand to grab my son.

I meant business and he knew it. Recognizing that I had control of the situation, he started walking away. Head down as a defeated animal, he left leaving the door opened behind him. Still holding my son, I quickly shut and locked the door. I grabbed a chair and secured it below the doorknob. Miraculously, my son slept through the whole ordeal. I put him back to bed.

It was time for me to go to bed. I was exhausted. I set my alarm for 7:00 am and just sat on my bed. I realized that my body was uncontrollably shaking. Staring into the dark, I held myself tightly and listened to the silence.

Tomorrow is a new day, the silence said.

The next day, I filed for divorce, with a restraining order. Since I was working as a legal secretary for an attorney, my boss called my husband and warned him to stay away from me or else he would be arrested immediately.

Although he had been warned before and being shocked by the eminent pending divorce, my husband suffered a sudden nervous breakdown and was hospitalized the following day. How ironic! I thought. You caused the pain and you are the one in the hospital.

He soon called and begged me to visit him with our son.

I wouldn't hear of it. Request denied! No more begging, crying and unkempt promises. Staying away from him was my only salvation, strength and my power.

Abuse is not okay!

Are you involved in an abusive relationship? If you are, pick up the phone right now and dial your way to freedom. There is help available today.

GETTING DIVORCED – 22 YEARS OLD

A preliminary court date settlement was scheduled three months after I filed for the divorce.

In the meantime, no provision was made to get any help from my husband, until that date. It was very difficult for me financially. I was barely making ends meet each month.

I was under a lot of stress most of the time and became sick. After the birth of my son, I developed painful bleeding hemorrhoids that needed to be surgically removed. In addition, my doctor had discovered a suspicious tumor, the size of a grapefruit, located inside the uterus and cysts on one of my ovaries. I was in pain most of the time. A date was set for the removal of my three bodily offenders.

Unfortunately, the surgery was scheduled to be done a week after the court hearing. I had to find someone to take care of my son, because I was to be hospitalized for a minimum of a week. In those days, that's how long you remained in the hospital after surgery, sometimes longer, depending on the procedure to be done.

I was already at the point of exhaustion, and my doctor's recommendation was to rest at home for at least one month after the surgery. I didn't have the money to pay for a 24-hour babysitter and my calls for help to friends and family remained unsuccessful.

Court day

Unlike my mother, my mother-in-law was more than willing to be my son's full time caretaker. My husband was living with his parents in a village some twenty miles away from the town that I was living in. My child would be taken care of until I would be able to return to work, a month after the surgery. And then, what I feared the most…happened.

As it turned out and against my desire, the court granted the temporary custody to my husband.

I was devastated! It was so unfair! My husband, with a smirk on his face, victoriously looked at me and said, "I told you, you would pay for what you did."

Do you see how twisted this is? This is how abusers will justify and continue to do what they do. In my husband's mind, he was now a victim and I had to pay for it.

Defeated and heartbroken, I left the court. I could hardly believe that after the record of verbal abuse and threats, the judge had so nonchalantly overlooked evidence of an unfit father and gave him temporary custody. This is another reason why abuse is allowed to continue in our society. Justice does not always prevail. In the early 70's, women were still considered inferior to men, regardless. Abuse was often ignored and tolerated.

Return to work

After my surgery, I was determined to get my son back as soon as possible. Against my doctor's advice, I immediately went back to work in order to contest the temporary custody.

It was a very dark period for me. Still weakened physically and emotionally, out of nowhere, I would burst into tears and just couldn't stop. I didn't like the world I was living in. It was cruel and unjust! Pure and simple, I felt victimized.

Adding to my antagonistic perspective of the human nature was the fact that I was working with my boss on a major criminal case. He was the defense attorney of a very highly sensitive and visible murder. His political career depended on this successful defense.

A seventeen year old girl had been kidnapped, raped, tortured and murdered. She was found naked in a ravine. I had seen pictures of her body darkened with bruises and cuts. She had long brown wet hair, with blood in it from a blow to her head. How could anyone do such a thing? It was horrific!

When I was called into the attorney's office to take stenographic dictation, the suspect was often present. He gave me the shivers! I couldn't help but think "Am I in the presence of a murderer?" The pictures were haunting me. I hated my boss for defending the suspect and I hated men for their violent behaviors and cruelty they directed toward women and children. Ultimately, I also hated myself for being involved in an abusive relationship.

On a side note, due to a lack of evidence, the suspect was acquitted and the murderer was never found. Case closed!

I was living in a very small town. I often thought that someone must have known something but kept quiet. Why?

Have you ever witnessed a crime? Or do you know of someone who did? What did you do? Did you keep quiet? Why?

Unexpected visit

One day, while at work, I was called to the front desk. My mother-in-law was in the waiting room with my son who was sleeping on her shoulder. I hadn't seen my little boy in two months. My husband made sure of that. The waiting room was filled with clients. Surprised and overwhelmed with emotions, I grabbed my son and moved away from watching eyes. It was raining outside and his little green jacket was wet. I grabbed my sweater from my chair and wrapped it around him. I gently kissed his face and his eyes that were still closed. I missed him so!

Holding my tears, I was almost choking. My mother-in-law followed me and said "I just have a few minutes. I have to go now," looking at me with tears in her eyes. She was a mother. She knew what I was feeling. As she was trying to take him back, he suddenly opened his eyes and with a stunned look, he exclaimed, "Maman!" Wrapping his little arms around my neck and putting his face against mine, I could no longer hold back my tears. "We have to go now" urgently said his grandmother, while trying to move him away from me. "NO! NO!" my son screamed, holding me tighter.

I wanted to run away with him and keep him safe and warm, but I knew that I had to let him go. Trying to be brave, I unwrapped his arms from around my neck and gave him back to his grandma. Forcefully, she was trying to hold him against her, as he was screaming and kicking with all his might. But... like a thief, she took him away. All was left of him was his shoe that fell off while he was fighting to stay with me. Exploding in tears, I bent over to pick it up. I looked up. He was gone. I held his shoe in the middle of my chest as if it were the last piece of him left.

Back in court

Considering that I had been back at work for two months, a new court date had been set. In a couple of weeks, I would be in front of the judge again. In the meantime, desperately wanting to start a new life with my son, I moved into a new apartment. I could hardly wait to have him back. In my new home, there was a play area filled with new toys. His bedroom was decorated in happy colors of green and blue and yellow. I had bought him new pajamas and bath bubbles. We needed to laugh again. He was about eighteen months old.

9:00 am. Outside the courtroom and seated on a bench while I waited, I saw my husband walking up to me. Defiantly he said, "You will never get him back." Simultaneously, my attorney opened the door of the courtroom and announced, "It's our turn now. Come in." This time, I felt confident. I was working and no longer sick. I looked at the new judge in front of me. His kind eyes reassured me and I felt safe. I took a deep breath and heard his irrevocable judgment, "With the new evidence presented to the court, the mother here and present, is given full custody of her son and will receive a monthly child support of $60."

I knew my son was waiting outside of the courtroom with his grandmother, at my attorney's request. I couldn't wait and ran outside the court. He was on the floor playing with a small toy. "Ross!" I screamed. As he looked up and saw me, he said "Oh maman," as he ran towards me. I picked him up, and victoriously declared, "We are going home now."

My son loved his new home and toys. We celebrated that night with ice cream and the new bubbles. They still made him laugh. I securely put him to bed and sang the lullaby that I used to sing for him. My treasure was back.

Provided that his father would pay child support, he was allowed monthly visits of one weekend a month. He came twice to pick him up. Then, still determined to get revenge, he stopped paying child support. I had to file a court order to seize his salary. Being obliged to pay, he stopped working. I had no more recourse to get the child support payments. I definitely was on my own.

MOVING AND CHANGING MY LIFE

My salary was not sufficient to support my son and myself. If I had unexpected expenses, it was very difficult to recover. Sometimes, I had to borrow canned food from my friend across the street for dinner. I had to find a better solution.

My sister Yvanne had just moved to Quebec City, 350 miles away and a place where we both dreamed of living. She called me one day to let me know of an opening in an attorney's office. I scheduled an appointment and drove the 350 miles for the interview. I got a job offer on the spot, with a catch. There was only a small increase in salary. My only hope was that once I moved there, I could find better opportunities. For that reason, I accepted the position.

Two weeks later, I was all settled in my new apartment and started my new job. Life was more expensive in Quebec. The day care was very costly. I was constantly juggling finances in my mind. Yvanne, who was a hairstylist, shared with me that one of her clients was making quite a bit of money working as a cocktail waitress in a discotheque. And apparently, they were hiring. I decided to check it out.

The disco was named *Rasputin,* after the historical Russian figure. Obviously, the Russian theme was very exotic. The cocktail waitresses were dressed in very striking attire. The place was electrifying! The music, the décor, the lights and the red couches were all strategically placed around the room to convey sensuality. Everyone, starting from the bus boy, to the barmaids, cocktail waitresses, disc jockey, and the doorman were absolutely gorgeous! Constant, the doorman was the sexiest man alive…after Elvis Presley. There was no doubt about that! It was so captivating to be in the disco era of the early 70's.

I definitely saw the potential of making a lot of money the first night that Yvanne and I checked it out. The place was jammed packed, with as many people inside as outside, waiting for the privilege to go in. I quickly made up my mind. "I will become a cocktail waitress," I told Yvanne. It was the solution to my financial problems.

It happened so fast. I could hardly believe it. I got hired. I felt pretty uncomfortable with the idea of wearing the see through mini dress, but I was willing to compromise, to lessen my monetary burdens. After all, I was not naked. I rationalized. Underneath the black silky dress, I was wearing a black bra and black panties. I would adjust; I convinced myself. I had to.

Have you ever comprised yourself to make more money? Not specifically, in the way that I did or perhaps in a even worse way. Look back and think of the ways you may have done it? Maybe you're doing it right now. Are you fully aware of all the ways you may be compromising some of your values to keep that job or to please your boss?

My first night

To complement my mini see-through dress, I wore four-inch high white shiny disco boots. A Russian flair was added by wearing a beautiful black fur hat. "Oh my," said co-worker Suzanne, looking at me in the mirror of the dressing room. "Looking pretty sexy tonight," she said, trying to make me relax. "Let's go practice. I have a few things to show you," she added and grabbed my arm.

In the center of the disco, there was a circular bar attended by three barmaids. The first in rank was a slim, stunning 5'11" blonde goddess with curly long hair down to her waist. Murielle was Constant's favorite. She had been there the longest and always got the best paying clients. Constant, being the manager of the disco had also designated Murielle as his assistant. She was married and had a five year old son. At the opposite end of the bar was Carmen, the second in rank. She was also a very tall, attractive 5'8" girl with shoulder length red hair and overflowing breasts. Carmen dated a biker who came every night after work to pick her up. In the middle of the bar, third in rank was Carole, a 5'7" short haired-brunette. Carole was extremely pretty with beautiful green eyes and a smile that was worth a $10.00 tip.

Working on the floor were 4 other girls, including myself. Each one of us had designated sections. For my first night, I was assigned to help Suzanne in handling the overflow of clients coming in. Suzanne was a beautiful blonde who was sweet as could be, with a big heart and a huge smile. We became the best of friends and had a friendship that lasted many years.

Marcelle, was another co-worker. She had long, thick, jet black hair and was very gregarious. She loved to flirt with the customers. Simone was the voluptuous one, with beautiful white teeth and mysterious green eyes. Her beauty didn't reflect her lifestyle. She was living on the edge and eventually got fired because of her drug usage. Then there was me, gorgeous France…(just kidding). I had blonde shoulder length hair, blue eyes, and a pretty smile. We were all very hard workers. Our living depending on it. There was camaraderie between us. I never witnessed an argument with anyone. There was fairness and teamwork.

At the entrance of the disco was a platform with lights swirling around the disc jockey, who was dressed in a sexy white outfit with an open shirt. He was dancing to the beats of Donna Summer, the Bee Gees, Michael Jackson, and KC & the Sunshine Band, to name just a few.

I started out on a Friday night. It was so busy.

Suzanne showed me how to hold a tray above my head, since we had to walk through the crowd with the tray filled with beers and other drinks.

Before we officially opened, I practiced a few times until I was getting the hang of it, or so I thought.

I loaded my tray with at least eight beers to sell to clients that were coming in. I ventured out into the crowd, balancing the tray above my head. I had almost reached the area where we greeted the clients when someone accidentally bumped into me. The eight beers ended up on the top of my head and hat, and drizzled down everywhere. Embarrassed and looking like a wet cat, almost in tears, I returned to the bar.

Suzanne who saw what had just happened, came to my rescue and ordered a cognac from the barmaid. "Here, drink this," she said while wiping me down with napkins. "It's hard the first time, but you'll get used to it." I drank the double cognac while she was busy refilling my tray. "You have to be aggressive," she said. "Push the people out of the way with your feet. They'll move." Somehow, I made it through my first night. I was exhausted but happy. After counting my tips, in one night I had made $200.00.

After a couple of months of working two jobs, I was getting burned out. I quit my daytime job, since I was making enough money at the disco. I decided to move closer to work which also meant living closer to where Yvanne lived. I bought an almost new Volvo. I was finally doing well.

NEW JOB AND NEW HUSBAND

Almost a year later, a new hotel that was being built attracted my attention. At the disco, I was working 6 days a week, very late hours and didn't see my son very much. The job was also very physically demanding. I interviewed for the opening at the new hotel as hostess/cocktail waitress and got the job. The hours were better. I had two days off and the atmosphere was sophisticated and elegant. I loved my new attire. I wore a beautiful long gold gown with a slight décolleté, with long sleeves and a discreet slit in the middle, from the bottom to approximately twelve inches above the knees. No more boots… but beautiful sandals. And I was twenty-five years old.

The bar was adjacent to a very elegant dining room on the twenty-fourth floor, with windows giving majestic views of the city and the Saint-Lawrence River. Jean-Louis, the maitre D was from Paris. Between the bar and the dining room area, was a platform for musicians to perform and a dance floor. The marketing approach of the hotel was to appeal to an international clientele. For that reason, an Italian guitarist and performer who sang in seven languages was hired to entertain on opening night.

Up to this point, five years after my divorce, my life had been consumed mainly with work and spending time with my son as much as I could. To the exception of a short dating period before I moved to Quebec, I had not been involved in a relationship.

Little did I know that on opening night, I was going to meet my second husband. He was the total opposite of my first husband. He had class and elegance. He was educated and well-versed. He also spoke French with a very pronounced Italian accent. He was good looking, had dark hair, brown eyes, very energetic, and sexy looking. There was no doubt in my mind. He was a charmer and a lady's man. The women, both young and old, loved him.

I was reluctant to accept an invitation to dinner. After all, his contract agreement with the hotel was for a short term. His persistence in inviting me out prevailed. I agreed to go to dinner with him on my day off, as long as my son was also invited. That was our first date.

MY SECOND SON

A year later, we married and shortly after, I gave birth to my second son. We named him Tiamo, which means "I love you", in Italian. Tiamo, who now is thirty-seven years old, is a very talented award-winning singer, songwriter and very successful business entrepreneur. If you would like to meet him, please visit his website at www.TiamoMusic.com

Thankfully, the birth process with Tiamo was not as traumatic and painful as the first one. At eight centimeters, I received an epidural that relieved some of the pain. And this time, I was not alone. My husband was there with me for the whole twelve hours of labor, reading a book about the process of giving birth. He was also present in the delivery room, ready with the camera.

Tiamo's name had been formulated by his father and I on a plane trip back from Italy, celebrated over a glass of champagne. Tiamo was a gorgeous little one with brown hair, brown eyes, and was looking straight up at me and the world when he was born!

I remained with Tiamo in the hospital for a couple of days. We bonded throughout the night, as he needed to be fed every two hours. He embodied a kind and gentle spirit. At the same time, he felt strong…as his little hand would hold on so tight to my finger while I was feeding him. He was already so aware, as he kept looking into my eyes while I gently hummed a song to him. When his hunger was satisfied, he would fall back into a deep sleep, with his head resting on my breast and his little mouth still open. I thought, *this is what peace looks like*. Tiamo was in total tranquility in my arms, held securely against my heart, without any need for anything else but the drifting away to a land of serenity. Sometimes, I would join him in that peaceful land. One of my favorite photos of us was captured that way—mother and son, eyes closed and mouths opened into restfulness and bliss.

There was a big celebration the night of Tiamo's entrance into the world. With half of his heritage being Italian, his grandmother came from Italy, one month prior to the birth. Tiamo was the first and only grandson in the family. She remained with us for three months after the birth. I loved her dearly. I knew enough Italian to communicate with her, since it was the only language she spoke. She was a kind, compassionate, wise and good-hearted woman. She totally dedicated her life to her family. Needless to say, she was filled with excitement when her son returned home and announced the arrival of her grandson. Our mutual friends also joined in the celebration and brought cigars and wine over.

My oldest son often told me that those family moments in the chalet in Lake Beauport were the happiest moments of his childhood. Finally there was a sense of unity. I will never forget the day when Ross held Tiamo in his arms and Tiamo laughed out loud for the first time. It was as though Tiamo had reserved that laughter specifically for his big brother. Ross was so happy and moved that he cried.

Life has a way of capturing these moments in time that are never erased from our memories.

That moment in time was the first gift they gave each other. Although they had different fathers, *they were brothers linked with the same heart—both giving and receiving in one instant, the joy of being together.*

MOVING TO ANOTHER COUNTRY

Six months after Tiamo's birth, we decided to move from the harsh winters of Quebec to the hot sun of Arizona. We left Canada in the month of February, during the blizzard of the century. When we landed in Arizona, I felt as though I had arrived in paradise. It was a beautiful, sunny, seventy-five degrees day. I was amazed by the majestic palm trees, the cacti, and the tall mountains shaped like *papier-mâché*, alternatively used in the English language as *paper mache*.

My husband's friends came to greet us upon arrival. Bob and Gail had pre-selected a furnished townhouse for us to move into. It was located in Scottsdale, in front of a pretty lake and park. Their daughter, Stephanie was my older son's age, which was seven years old. They became very good friends and went to school together. Gail and I immediately connected and became best friends, despite the language barrier. Bob was my husband's partner in business. Together they started a booking agency for musicians.

Many adjustments had to be made, including a new language for my son and I to learn, a new culture, and we were away from everything and everyone we had ever known. Before leaving Quebec, I had a last dinner with my family that was filled with deep emotions. My parents had come to visit me in Quebec and so did Regine, who lived in Montreal at the time. She was married and pregnant with her first child. Yvanne, still living in Quebec, was in a serious relationship. It was difficult to move so far away, not knowing when we would see each other again. It was especially difficult for Yvanne and me, since we had never been apart from one another.

But I knew that there was a new and exciting life in front of me. I was filled with hope for the future. I was twenty-eight years old and I was fearless.

I remained in Arizona for thirty-three more years.

Taking much longer than anticipated for the business to take off, my husband contacted his agent to get booking engagements for live performances again. Then, an opportunity came up and my husband had to leave for Connecticut for six months. With the savings being depleted, we agreed that I would help out and look for a job.

I saw an ad for a portrait consulting agency called PCA International. The job offered a base salary plus commission. I got hired and was set to start the following month, after the completion of the studios that were being built in four different areas. The consultants had to navigate between the four studios.

In the meantime, my sister Yvanne had come to visit me. She was not doing well emotionally and was drinking quite heavily. Scotch on the rocks was her drink of choice. Pretty tipsy one evening, she revealed to me the reason for her visit. She was heartbroken. Her boyfriend of almost two years left her. She didn't feel that life was worth living and she had come to see me and the children for the last time.

I was aware of her depressive state since we often spoke on the phone, but I didn't know the severity of it. Yvanne was very good at pretending and covering up her real emotional state. Not that night however. "I miss you so much and the kids," she said. "You are my family. I feel so alone and I can't stand it. I came to say goodbye and I'm going to end this agony." Very alarmed, I knew that if she was to go back to Canada, I risked losing her forever. I had to find a solution. I adored my sister! Lying in bed that night, I found the answer.

Over coffee the next morning, I announced, "Darling sis, this is what we are going to do, and keep in mind that what I am about to tell you is not open for discussion." Surprised by my firm tone, she sat back in her chair and intensely looked at me with her big blue hangover eyes.

The plan: Saving Yvanne's life

Lighting up an extra long Virginia Slims cigarette, I declared, "I am starting a new job in a few weeks and I will need a babysitter. Ross is in school until 3:00 pm and you will take care of Tiamo while I go to work. You will stay here with me. I will feed you and will provide whatever you need until you get established here." "But, France that's not possible" she interjected. Ignoring her, I continued, "We will call Regine in Montreal and ask her to sell your furniture and send you the money. She will ship your clothes by train. You are not going back to Canada! As of today, this is your new home. You are staying here with us."

In disbelief, she stared at me without saying a word. But, I saw a light in her eyes. She had hope. "Oh my God" she said. "I don't even know a word of English and I am not legal here." "It will work out," I reassured her. "We'll figure it out, you'll see." "Okay" she said with a smile. "I agree."

I knew I was going to have my hands full. But, it was a necessary move. It would change her life. And on the subject of changing her life, I came up with another plan. In order to help her through her depression, I took her to see a therapist. The only problem was that Yvanne didn't speak or understand a word of English. After making proper arrangements with the therapist, we agreed that I would translate the conversation back and forth between the two of them. At first, we went twice a week. Slowly, she started feeling better.

A few months had gone by and one major obstacle remained unsolved. She didn't have legal status in the U.S. However, the solution would later appear to me after one evening when Yvanne, Gail and I decided to go out dancing and have fun.

It was a Saturday night and the club was jamming. The band was playing the famous song by The Platters "Only You" when Rob, a stunning looking man, asked Yvanne to dance. It was love at first sight, or should I say attraction at first sight—love being a total different thing. Since Yvanne's knowledge of English was still extremely limited, he asked my permission to take Yvanne on a date the following night. I agreed to let her go on the condition that he gave me his driver's license number and car registration information when he came to pick her up the following evening. Their love affair started.

Although there was much translation needed when they were together, they got along well enough, and that's when I found the solution to legalize Yvanne in the U.S. In agreement with Yvanne, I asked Rob to marry her. That way, she would become a legal resident. I thought that they could always get divorced later on, if the marriage didn't work out. Rob agreed, and six months later, they were married and moved into a house that Rob had just purchased as an investment.

The suicide attempt

Rob was very busy trying to make money in real estate, refurbishing homes and reselling them. He was constantly working until late in the evenings. Yvanne was sitting at home, bored to death. Lonely, she drank even more every night. She knew that she had a huge problem, but she didn't want to stop. "It's helping me cope," she said to me one night.

On the contrary, the drinking aggravated her depression.

One day, I received a call from Rob. "Yvanne took a bunch of pills. They are taking her right now to the emergency room. Can you come?" Rob asked. When I got to the hospital, she was in the ICU, hooked up to tubes and oxygen. She was lying there, pale and almost lifeless. The doctors were still pumping her stomach as I saw a very dark grayish liquid coming out through a tube inserted in her mouth. "She may not survive," I was told by the doctors. They were doing everything they could.

She was thirty years old. This was her second suicide attempt. The first one was five years earlier in Canada. She had left a note for Rob that said, "It's not your fault." Rob had come home earlier that day and found her almost breathless on the bedroom floor. Overwhelmed that night he told me, "I can't take care of her anymore. You need to take over or I'll put her somewhere." When I found out that putting her somewhere meant in a mental hospital, outraged, I replied, "How dare you! Yes, she needs help, but to put her away in a mental hospital is pushing it. After this crisis is over with, I'll decide what will be best to do."

I had no idea what I was going to do. She had been in Intensive Care for three days and she was still unconscious. All I could do was to wait. On the fourth day, I received a call. Broken up on the phone was Yvanne's voice. "France, can you come, please?" I drove so fast to the hospital. I was hysterically laughing and crying at the same time. They had moved her from the ICU, and now, she was alive and speaking! I held her in my arms while caressing her hair. "I am so sorry, France" she said. "I know," I replied.

After speaking to her doctor, I was extremely relieved to find out that there was no evidence of brain damage. Upon release from the hospital, she had to follow up with a psychiatrist and continued with the prescribed medication to ease the symptoms of her severe depression.

After a few weeks, Yvanne decided to enter a detoxification program in a specialized hospital. She remained there for two weeks and continued with a 12-step program afterwards. She was slowly gaining some inner strength and was no longer at the mercy of her addiction. I was very proud of her.

Building a brand new life

Despite Yvanne's progress, one major question remained. How could she be in control of her own life without being completely dependent on her husband? After speaking with Rob, he agreed to buy Yvanne a used car. "And I'll teach her how to drive," I had said. On my days off, we practiced driving the car and together, we studied the driver's license book. She passed the written and driving tests with flying colors. She was so proud of herself. The car had given her much more freedom and she enjoyed going to the 12-step program as often as she wanted. She met some new people and made friends. They understood her. She had a sponsor that was available twenty-four hours a day, in case she needed help.

She was connecting with the world again. Rob was feeling much better and bought Yvanne a little white dog with curly hair. She named him "Bully." While Rob was busy working, she had a new companion to keep her company.

Next on the list was to help her in getting a job. She had a cosmetology license from Canada, but needed more hours for the U.S. licensing. Together, we studied the requirements and the new book in English. After six months, she was ready to take the test and got her license. All she had to do now was to get a job! And she did! Her life was looking up. She was happier. Although Rob was still a very busy man, she was feeling better and was slowly building her life without depending so much on him.

In the meantime, while she was reshaping her life, my life had taken another turn. Shortly after moving to Arizona, I found out that my husband had been unfaithful to me. For a few months, I went to therapy. He came with me a few times, but was mostly out-of-town with his job requirements. I often went alone. I was working on my own self-esteem issues and in the process, I had decided to give my husband another chance.

Several months later, chance would have it that a letter addressed to him was delivered at our home, instead of his office. The feminine envelope and return address raised suspicion inside of me. My heart was beating out of my chest. I found out that he was having an affair with someone else in Connecticut. Unable to remain faithful to me, I filed for divorce. My youngest son was two years old and my oldest was nine. Although the divorce was painful for both of us we mutually agreed to maintain a close friendship and so we did for over 30 years now. Not only did we keep in contact but Franco, Tiamo's father always made sure that he would see his son whom he loved dearly as often as he could in spite of his heavy travels around the world. He also kept a close relationship with my oldest son which I am very grateful for. He cared for him as his own son and always made a point of keeping in touch with him throughout the years. That link built over 30 years ago has never been broken between the three of us.

However, back in time I found myself at a crossroads again. I was fighting my own battles of depression and anxiety. Although my husband was paying child support, I was not making the same amount of money as before. The company I worked for had been sold, and the bonuses were eliminated. In addition, the commission had been lowered as well. I had to find a better paying job. Going back to the newspapers ads again, I noticed that two full pages were dedicated to programmer/analyst positions, with a good starting salary. I decided that I would become a programmer/analyst.

Going to college at 32 years old

We sold the townhouse that my husband and I owned in Scottsdale and my children and I *moved to Tucson, Arizona* where I would attend college. Two years later, I graduated with honors. Since I only had a degree and no experience, I started working as a computer operator on the third shift, from midnight to 8:00 am. IBM, my employer, had hired me for a six-month temporary job. This was not the dream job I had studied for, but I needed work, so I accepted the position. I had no idea was I was in for.

All the reports were printed at night on several, eight feet long IBM printers. There were three of them spiting paper out all night long, plus two other printers dedicated to special forms. Every load of paper taken off from the printer had to be separated and loaded into boxes. I had to take those heavy boxes down the steps from the printing room into a designated bin area where a courier would pick them up in the morning. It was a very physically demanding job. Nothing had prepared me for this type of work. I couldn't adjust to the crazy hours and was getting very little sleep during the day. After the six-month period was over, I moved back to Phoenix for a job offer as a computer operator and I was going to work the second shift. "How could I ever get the programmer job I desperately wanted?" Ross was thirteen years old and Tiamo was six.

Mutilation

After three years living in Tucson, I was so happy to move back to Phoenix and be closer to my sister. Yvanne was still with Rob, working and sober. Some health issues had come up for her after a visit to her gynecologist, and she was told that she needed to have a hysterectomy. The news, although distressing, was not devastating to her. She didn't want children at that time and didn't foresee wanting any in the near future. She always said to me "I have your children, France. I feel as close to them as if they were mine." She indeed loved my children very much. She often told Ross, "I am your second mom."

Her surgery was successful. Although the doctors suspected cancer, the results were negative. In that same period of time, I started having very strange bleeding episodes. After tests and exams, my gynecologist couldn't find the source of the problem. I was left in the dark about what to do next. Later, Yvanne asked me "Why don't you get a hysterectomy, like I did? It will solve your problem," she added nonchalantly, as if we were talking about the removal of a tooth.

For many months, I lived in fear about not knowing the cause of the bleeding. Yvanne's suggestion seemed to be a feasible solution to my problem, even if it was a pretty extreme one. I went back to my gynecologist and suggested that option to him. In spite of the consequences that he made me aware of in proceeding with the surgery, I was amazed at how easy it was to convince him to perform it. Maybe the dollar signs had taken over his medical etiquette? He scheduled the surgery for the following month.

They removed everything—ovaries, uterus, the whole enchilada, gone! Strangely enough, my doctor told me that he had found a rare type of internal cyst that was causing the bleeding. All he had to do was to remove it and nothing else. But, since I had pushed for the whole surgery to be performed, in spite of finding the source of the bleeding, he proceeded anyway with the removal of all the organs. I found out later that my sister and I had developed the same rare condition. How strange! We both had unconsciously developed this bleeding disorder at the same time. According to Louise Hay, the interpretation of the probable cause of a cyst is "running the old painful movie." I believe that Yvanne and I had stored our childhood story in our bodies. I believe that if medicine would only deal with the root of the problem first, many illnesses could be alleviated, if not all of them.

Did you know that according to a survey done by the Centers for Disease Control and Prevention that approximately 600,000 hysterectomies are performed each year in the United States at an estimated annual cost of more than $5 billion? More than one-fourth of U.S. women will have this procedure done by the time they are 60 years of age.

Hysterectomy is the second most frequent major surgical procedure among reproductive-aged women.

Determination

After my recovery, I continued looking for work. It had been almost two years since my college graduation. Programming positions were still very much in demand, but work experience was required. How could I ever get the experience I needed, in order to be employed?

In the meantime, I was also looking for other positions to work first shift as a computer operator. Because of my work hours, I couldn't see my children very much and it was really hard on all of us. But then I had learned that a company called EDS was hiring for computer operators on all three shifts. I took the chance and went for an interview, specifically asking for the daytime position, not realizing that to be considered for employment, I had to be available for all three shifts.

A week after my interview, I called the manager to find out if I was considered for the position. He said, "Frankly, no France—the reason being that you are not flexible in working all three shifts, which means that I am forced to consider you only for the daytime position and that is not fair for the other applicants." "Please consider me for all three shifts" I replied immediately. "But keep in mind that first shift is my preference. Will you consider that?" I asked. "Well, yes I will" he replied.

Two days later, I called him back. "Have you made a decision?" I bravely asked. "No, not yet" he said. "We have many applicants to consider. I will let you know." "Mr. Gardner," I responded "Can you at least tell me if I am being considered for the position?" Laughing, he replied, "Well, yes". "Great, thank you very much" I said enthusiastically. Three days later, still no news. I called him again and he said, "I was going to call you today. We have three finalists for each shift. You belong to one of those categories. Can you come in for another interview?"

I had the second interview with Mr. Gardner, the manager of operations, and Alice, the immediate supervisor. It went really well. I knew I would get the job. The only thing I didn't know was for which shift I was being interviewed for. The reason why I wanted to be employed by this company was to have decent working hours so I could spend time with my sons. In addition, there were possibilities for me to finally move up to programming.

Two days later, still, no calls. "What was taking so long?" I impatiently asked myself. I called Mr. Gardner again and in one long sentence, I held my breath and asked, "Since you have selected the candidates for all three shifts already, no one objects to any shifts except me, you need someone to work the first shift, and I am the only one in need of those hours, can you just please tell me if I got the job?" And then, I relaxed when I heard a big laugh on the other end of the line. "I was prepared to make you a job offer today, but informally, before I put it on paper, would you like to work for us?" Then I asked, "For first shift?" Laughing even louder, he said, "We need people like you working for us. Your determination has been rewarded. Yes, first shift it is." "Yeah!" I exclaimed. "When can you start?" he asked. Two weeks later, I started my daytime job. Finally, I could be at home at decent hours and have more time with my children.

Meeting his father for the 1ˢᵗ time

Many times in the past, my oldest son requested to meet his father. I contacted him in Canada to let him know of my son's wish. We agreed that Ross would visit him during his summer school break. Ross was fourteen years old, at the time. Already, my son was dealing with many difficult issues as a teenager. In retrospect, it was a terrible time for both of them to meet. And when Ross came back home from visiting his father, he was changed, confused, and very resentful towards me. The bond and closeness we always shared had been brutally shaken. My son's strong desire to identify with his father led to him rebelling against me.

Suddenly, we became rivals. He was defying my authority and I was lost on what to do. For support, I joined a tough love parenting group and I applied their philosophy. Many parents had very good results, and that was encouraging. Unfortunately, after many unsuccessful trial and error cycles and three years of ongoing conflict between us, it was decided that it would be best for my son to go to Canada and stay with his father. All of my life, I had fought so hard to keep him and in the process, I overcame any and all obstacles in front of me—except this one. We were no longer fighting together to survive, but against each other. We had to separate. He remained with his father a few months and eventually moved to Montreal, Canada where he started his own journey.

Throughout his life, Ross overcame many hardships. He put himself through college and he is now a very successful Systems Analyst working for a prominent bank in Canada. I am extremely proud of him! We overcame many difficult challenges from the past, as it took a lot of love and forgiveness on both sides.

Sadly, we lost many years trying to fix an old bridge that was leading us in different directions. Today, we are building a new bridge, and together, we are walking hand in hand toward a beautiful new pathway that is opening up in front of us. Now, there is no more suffering, no more ruptures, and no more broken hearts. We did that way too much before. By building a bridge with the pillars of love, we are sure to reach a peaceful shore together. The love we always had for each other cannot fail us.

Just recently, I was reflecting on how major life events repeat themselves through our children. I left home when I was seventeen years old, so did Ross. I went to college and became a system analyst, so did he. And, we just realized a few months ago that we both bought our first home at the same age.

And life goes on…

After eight years of marriage, Yvanne filed for divorce. She was still sober, had her own place, and was doing well at work. After the divorce, her emotions were shaky, but manageable. She was still getting a lot of support from the AA group that she belonged to, from her friends, and from me.

At this point, I had been working at EDS for almost two years and there were still no openings in the programming department. It was time to go back to the "good old friend of mine", the newspaper. "Surely, a programmer trainee position would open up one day," I thought.

Moving again and my new job

On Sunday mornings, Tiamo and I had a ritual. We loved to go out for donuts. Over coffee and orange juice, we religiously ate our freshly baked chocolate donuts. We talked about fun things like his friends and music. He was playing the flute in school and played the piano at home. He talked about his passion, basketball, and his best friend Joey. We often laughed about nothing. I'm sure that sugar had a lot to do with it. Sometimes after donuts, we would go for a Sunday drive. Many times, while Tiamo played outside, I submerged myself in the newspaper to look for jobs and send my resume to potential employers.

On one of those Sundays, a newspaper ad attracted my attention. It was for a programmer analyst position with a minimum of two years experience. It was a government job for Pinal County in Florence, Arizona. Where the heck was Florence, Arizona? Since the prospect of moving again didn't appeal to me, I threw away the newspaper. But, throughout the week, there was a little voice inside of me that said, "You need to reply to that ad." By Wednesday, I heard the voice even louder while I was driving home after work. I pulled the newspaper out of the trashcan. The ad was still intact. After I sealed the addressed white envelope containing my resume and cover letter, I felt a sense of relief. I mailed it the next morning on my way to work. The inner voice was satisfied.

On Monday of the following week, I received a call from the programming manager of Pinal County to schedule an interview. I left early from work the following day to meet with both the director of the data processing department and the manager. It was Thanksgiving week and very quiet in the office. I was greeted by a programmer and led into an office where the interview was conducted.

I had worn a wool grey and white suit for my interview. I was obviously overdressed. My interviewers were wearing sweaters and jeans. It was a very relaxed atmosphere. "I wish I could feel as relaxed inside," I thought.

Do you believe in divine coincidences? The main reason why I was contacted for the interview was that Ray, who was the director, recognized my name on the resume. I had been one of his students in college. As soon as we saw each other, we both recognized where we had met before. Ray was a very loud, gregarious, and expressive man. Jerry, the manager, was a very kind, nice looking, and soft-spoken man. He had a calming effect during the interview process. I felt at ease with both of them.

My lack of experience didn't seem to matter, as I felt they both liked me as well. Personality was more important to them than experience. Two days later, I received a call from Jerry. "When can you start?" he asked. "In two weeks," I gladly replied. "After I give my notice and find an apartment." Finally, I had the job I wanted! I was hired as a programmer analyst. I was willing to make sacrifices, which meant moving again and working in a very small town. I chose to live in Casa Grande, which had more to offer than Florence.

When I told Tiamo the following day about the move, understandably, he was not too happy. It meant losing his friends and changing schools. When we sat down and discussed the possibilities of liking his new school and making new friends, he changed his stance. "I will think about it," he said. "Let me know when you feel you are okay with my decision" I replied. I wanted to give him time to think on his own. The next day, he declared. "Mom, I am fine now. I am not upset anymore and I am okay to move." "I am very happy about that son, let's celebrate!" Over cookies and cream ice cream, we started making new plans. Tiamo was ten years old and I was turning thirty-nine that week.

That weekend, we went to Casa Grande and found an apartment we both liked. There was a pool, a playground, and plenty of kids playing outside. We moved in December. Another cycle had just begun. Little did I know, that I was going to meet my third husband.

PART 6

FROM 39 YEARS OLD TO PRESENT DAY

A PRELUDE TO MY NEW RELATIONSHIP JOHNNY AND REBECCA

"Come and play with me!" exclaimed Johnny the squirrel, to his squirrel friend Rebecca. "I really enjoy being with you. If you stay with me through the harsh winters, I'll give you all the nuts and seeds that you could ever need. I will keep you warm in the little house I built in the woods and protect you against any predators. I'll try to make you happy every day. And, you'll never need to go outside if you don't want to." "But, I like to go outside and play" Rebecca responded. "Okay, fair enough, as long as you come back to me." Johnny replied. "Well, I don't know if I want to move in with you" Rebecca hesitated. "I sure like you a lot, but I'm used to getting my own food and building my own house." "I know, but together we could learn about love" Johnny interjected. "Love?" questioned Rebecca.

"Yeah, that's the only thing I will ever need from you" Johnny affirmed. "You will have to love me more than anything in the world and tell me everyday" Johnny continued. "And why do I have to do that?" Rebecca asked, puzzled. "Because I don't know what love feels like and I want that feeling, above all else." "I think I know what you're talking about, Johnny. I heard all the other squirrels talking about it the other day. They called it a feeling, but no one knows how to find it. It sure seems to be elusive around here! And you Johnny, what do you know about it?" Rebecca asked, intrigued by Johnny's proposal. "Well, from the latest I heard on the subject, you need to have a heart to get it." "A heart?" replied Rebecca. "Yeah" replied Johnny. "When you have a heart, which we have, you can receive love" Johnny responded. "But how?" Rebecca questioned, unconvinced. Frustrated by his lack of knowledge, Johnny simply replied, "Well, you have to hear words of love from another squirrel. And that's how love gets put into your heart. So, you see Rebecca, by being together, we can tell each other those words." "Oh!"

62

exclaimed Rebecca. "That's how it works huh! Well, that seems easy enough. Let's give it a try."

And so, Rebecca moved in with Johnny. Every day, Rebecca told Johnny how much she loved him and Johnny did the same for Rebecca. And some months later, their neighbor Sam came over to borrow a few seeds. "Hey buddy, how is it going Johnny? I have company tonight; can I borrow a few seeds from you?" Sam asked. "Sure" Johnny gladly obliged, already fixing a seed-to-go bag. "By the way, Johnny, are you getting that love you wanted?" Sam curiously asked. Unable to answer, Johnny looked down on the floor and replied impatiently, "You better get going. I have things to do now." Unhappy and needing to fill the void that Johnny felt in his heart, he sat down and opened a bag of nuts. He didn't want to tell Sam or even admit to himself that despite hearing Rebecca's words of love, he still did not feel it inside of him like he thought he would. Disappointed and irritated, he blamed Rebecca for not giving him the love he so desired. She did her best to convince him, but realized that it was useless. She felt discouraged and wanted to give it up. "That love stuff is not getting into our hearts," she sadly admitted to Johnny. "What's the use? You don't believe me anyway, Johnny." So, she stopped telling Johnny what he wanted to hear, and instead, she told him how unhappy she felt. And, Johnny did the same.

But, Johnny didn't want Rebecca to leave, so he tried to make her smile and laugh again. When she didn't, he became angry and said hurtful words that made her cry. He felt bad for doing that, but he couldn't help himself. "Why can't I get what I want?" he cried out to her one day.

Resentful and depressed, Rebecca withdrew into herself. "Why is this "love" so evasive and mysterious?" she pondered. Every squirrel I know is either miserable, or looking for it, or unable to find it. Even the ones that say they have it seem gloomier after they realize that it's not what they thought it would be.

One day while packing a bag of nuts, Rebecca announced, "I have to go Johnny. I must leave and find my own answers. When I find out what love is, I'll come back and let you know all about it." With tears in her eyes, Rebecca quickly opened the door and left.

Many months later, Rebecca was exploring a nearby lake and saw a woman sitting on a bench close to her. The woman opened up a bag and put some food on the ground. Hungry, Rebecca approached the bench to pick it up. "My, what's that?" asked Rebecca. "Hi there, it's a cookie" answered the woman. "A cookie? It's mighty delicious!" exclaimed Rebecca, holding it between her claws. "Glad you like it" the woman happily replied.

"What's that you're holding?" Rebecca curiously asked. "Oh, that's a book" replied the Woman. "Do tell more, please" invited Rebecca. "Well, a book is a story that someone has written and others read for enjoyment." "That sounds like fun! What's the story about?" Rebecca asked. "It's a love story" the woman said. "A what? Did you say love? Like in L.O.V.E?" exclaimed Rebecca, with her mouth wide open, dropping the rest of the cookie on the ground. As good as that cookie was, nothing was more important in that moment than what Rebecca wanted to hear. "Come and sit by me," the woman

said. *"Do you want to learn about love?"* she gently probed Rebecca. *"Are you kidding me? For such a long time, I have been searching for answers. Is this something you can teach me?"* wished Rebecca. *"Well, I hope so. Maybe I can help."* The woman replied. *"Oh yes, ma'am, I do want to know everything about it"* Rebecca cried out, still in disbelief about her luck—first the cookie, and now she finally could learn something about love! "I can't wait to tell Johnny" Rebecca thought to herself.

And so, the woman started reading the love story to Rebecca. After giving her a condensed version of the first two chapters, she read her the third one—the final chapter... the one that Rebecca would find the answers that she was seeking. Rebecca would discover the path to LOVE.

"Envision this Rebecca," the woman continued...

A SOUL AGREEMENT

"Envision a past life soul agreement between two weary travelers from different parts of the world, landing in the same airport and arriving at the exact same checkpoint" the woman said to Rebecca as she warmly invited her into her story. "Imagine a security officer, commanding the two to open their suitcases. Simultaneously, the travelers lay down their suitcases and opened them for the officer.

The two travelers can't help but glance at each other's bags that lay side by side during the inspection. Both travelers are stunned when they realize that they are carrying similar contents—wounds from childhood, failed marriages, comparable careers, children, and unhealed stories from their past.

"What's inside this package?" demands the officer, picking up a wrapped gift. "As you can see officer, it is meant to be opened by the one who will know my heart, as it is inscribed on the ribbon" says the male traveler. "Oh! I have the same ribbon!" the other traveler enthusiastically declares. Amazed, they look at each other. They already know what's inside the wrapped package—hope, compassion, kindness, courage, devotion, sensitivity, joy, determination, commitment, and love.

"How could this be possible?" they whisper to each other. "Very well" interrupts the officer. "That will do. Move along now. Next in line please." Immediately after the checkpoint, the travelers have to separate and go off in different directions. "How will I recognize you when we meet again in the human world, since we won't remember the pre-birth agreement between our souls?" she asks him as they close their suitcases. "Your hands" he responds. "I will recognize your hands" as he watches her closing her suitcase. "I already know your heart."

So, that's how it all began—on that November day, when they met again. As he had promised her, he recognized her first. He was entranced by the look of her hands, gently sitting on her lap during a job interview. "Where do I know her from?" he silently questioned himself.

So months later, the night they danced and kissed, they recognized the gift wrapped with the scripted ribbon. "I know your heart" he undoubtedly told her. "And so do I" she replied.

In that mutual recognition, they found each other again. Now, with a new journey ahead, they moved into discovering each other and most of all, themselves, the woman concluded with Rebecca.

Their common background

One of the traveler's names is Jerry. He was born in Michigan with blond hair and green eyes. His father, whom he never met, was a drug addict and an alcoholic. He had a violent temper and often physically abused Jerry's mother. Thankfully for him, Jerry's parents got divorced when he was still a baby. His father died of a drug overdose at the age of thirty-one. Jerry was raised by his grandmother, whom he dearly loved. He often told me that his grandma and I shared the same kindred spirit. Jerry's mother remarried when he was five years old. Abruptly, Jerry was removed from the care of his grandma to live with his mom and her new husband. From that union, two girls were born. Jerry recalls his mother as being cold and unloving toward him. In her dating days before this marriage, she often told Jerry "Don't call me Mom when you see me with someone. Call me Betty."

At nineteen, Jerry got married to a beautiful girl of the same age. They moved to California that same year. A son was born the following year and three daughters followed. Their marriage lasted eighteen years. Jerry was very unhappy and filed for divorce. He got remarried two years later and moved to Tucson, Arizona. Two years later, he divorced again. His wife was unfaithful.

I, the other traveler, was born to an abusive alcoholic father. I didn't feel loved by him. My mother was not an affectionate woman. I also had two sisters. At five years old, I was sent to live in the orphanage. Like Jerry, I got married at nineteen. I gave birth to my first son the following year. That marriage ended in divorce two years later. I remarried seven years later, and divorced for the second time two years later. My husband was unfaithful.

So there we were! Both of us derived from similar backgrounds with abusive, addictive, unloving parents. In addition, we both were married at a very young age and were the primary caretakers of our children. We got divorced twice and worked in data processing, which we didn't like, but it served the purpose of financially surviving. We lived almost identical scripts.

After living two similar yet very separate lives, we arrived at the same destination, in the same year, in the same small western town with a total population of 4,000 people, in 1987. Coincidence or pre-destination?

As the manager, Jerry often organized social group outings such as picnics, camping trips and going to musical theater shows. I had been working with Jerry for six months, when one day, out of the blue, he asked me out to dinner. Since he was a very kind, fun and spirited man, I accepted the invitation.

Considering my preferences for seafood and filet mignon, Jerry selected an upscale restaurant in the Phoenix area that offered both. After dinner and a lively conversation over a bottle of wine, we agreed to go dance the night away.

Jerry was a bit tense on the dance floor. To ease the awkwardness, I laughingly said "I think you need to relax a little. Have fun with the music!" Unexpectedly, Jerry held my face between his hands and kissed me. In that moment, it's as though we recognized each other. It was a déjà vu experience from that "checkpoint in the airport". As we slow-danced to the song "Lady In Red", he whispered in my ears "I know your heart."

After that, everything moved so fast! On our third date, Jerry declared his love for me: "I have never met anyone like you" he said looking into my eyes. "You are kind, loving and compassionate. You have a great sense of humor and you find the deep values in people around you. I want to marry you."

At first, I was taken aback by the speedy proposal. It was too fast for me. I felt extremely close to him, but I was not ready for marriage. "Let's take it easy for now" I responded. "Let's see where this romance take us, okay?" "Of course" he responded. "I only want you to know how deep my feelings are for you."

The small town of Florence, Arizona, where I was employed had little, to no opportunities for career advancement. After a year, I applied for a better paying job in the metropolitan area of Phoenix. After a successful third interview, I received a job offer and moved back to Phoenix. Jerry came to visit on weekends, while he was seeking a management position in the city. Eventually, Jerry proposed again and this time, I said yes. We set a date for the wedding. Two years after we met and four days prior to my birthday in November, we were married. I was forty-one years old and Jerry was forty-five.

THE WEDDING AND THEREAFTER

Our wedding day was truly a fairy tale. Everything was absolutely perfect! I felt like a princess. The song my husband chose for our wedding dance was "One in A Million." "Honey, you are one in a million" he whispered in my ears. We were both dressed in white as if it was our first wedding. What a stunning couple we were!

Jerry's three daughters from California, his son from Seattle, and my oldest son from Canada came to Arizona for the occasion. Jerry's youngest daughter was my bridesmaid and my youngest son Tiamo, age thirteen, gave me away. A son, giving his mother away on her wedding day—what a beautiful love story! Twenty-three years later, life presented me with the opportunity to do the same for Tiamo, when he entered marriage on August 25, 2013.

Tiamo had selected a minister, a close friend of his, to perform his wedding ceremony. A day before the wedding, his friend cancelled and said that he couldn't make it to perform the wedding due to a family emergency. And that's when I got the surprising phone call. "Mom, you will never guess what just happened" Tiamo said to me on the phone. "What is it Tiamo?" "Well, my friend had an emergency and can't come to marry us. Would you perform our wedding ceremony?" "ME?!" I exclaimed in disbelief. "Yes Mom, I found out that you can apply to become a minister on the internet" he reassured me. "You can get a license up to twenty-four hours before the wedding" he continued. "Mom, I can't think of a better person than you to marry me tomorrow." "It will be my honor, son" I replied. I was extremely touched by his request. Looking at the clock, I exclaimed "Oh my God, we only have twenty-six hours left! I better get going."

The following day in, front of seventy very astounded guests, I performed the wedding ceremony!

Now, back to my wedding...

Holding Tiamo's arm, mother and son walked down the aisle. "Who gives this woman in marriage?" asked the minister. "I do" Tiamo proudly replied. Framed under an oval arch, filled with white and pink roses, Jerry and I exchanged our written vows. Adding to the tone of our words were the soft notes of the harp being played in the background and the slow movement of the water flowing from the outdoor fountain.

We exchanged red roses as the expression of our love. "When and if difficulties arise, and you are unable to speak" said the Minister, "Place a red rose for the other to see. It will serve as a reminder of the love and the commitment you both made to each other today." Hence, my nickname *Little Flower*, chosen by Jerry. Years later, he had an angel, holding a red rose tattooed on his right arm. The inscription reads "Little Flower."

Our wedding day was sunny and warm. And the following day was cold and rainy. The fairy tale was over. At the sound of the bell, Cinderella rushed back home to a life she didn't want to relive. In becoming a husband, Jerry put a lot of pressure on himself and assumed many roles. He wanted to be everything and all for me, so that I would never need anyone else in my life. Some of those roles were very positive in a marriage, but others created huge problems.

For instance, if at any moment I didn't seem "happy enough", he interpreted that as a personal defeat and that he was failing badly at being a good husband. The pressure was equally great on my side, as no one can possibly be happy and smiling all the time. Over breakfast one morning during our honeymoon, he said to me "You don't seem happy". What's wrong?" *Sound familiar?*

Combined with the sense of failure in achieving his multiple roles, his lack of self-love and self-esteem became explosive. I felt as though he was constantly trying to provoke a reaction in me that would confirm what he felt inside. I felt watched and often attacked. My husband was a mixture of a protector and a predator.

"You don't love me enough" became one of his favorite complaints. How extraordinary it is that when lacking self-love, one cries out to the other "you don't love me enough." That was illustrated when, while having dinner one evening during our honeymoon, he accused me of flirting with the waiter. I left the table, crying.

Jerry had difficulties trusting women, in general. The inability to love himself emphasized his growing fear of losing me. In an effort to prevent what he dreaded the most, he became very controlling and possessive. At the same time, he showered me with all he could give, so I would never want to leave. Of course, his efforts exhausted him and he became angrier.

"Why was this happening?" I desperately asked myself. "Why do I keep repeating the same patterns in my life?" I had seen warning signs before the wedding day. Why did I choose to go through it?

While dating Jerry, my counselor calmed my fears one day when she advised me, "Jerry's love for you will prevail. You both have much to overcome from the past" she continued. "But once Jerry learns to trust you, all his doubts will fade away." Reassured, I left her office that day, hoping that there was a good chance for our relationship to work out. As I drove home, I recalled all the good qualities Jerry had. He was kind, loving, and was a committed and devoted man. I decided to follow my counselor's advice. I never would have predicted what was to come.

Coming back from our honeymoon, we both yelled at each other "let's get a divorce!"

One day, Tiamo overheard our heated discussion. "Why do people get married, only to get divorced after" he said crying. "Why can't you work it out, Mom?" Wiping his tears, I replied "I'll work it out, Tiamo."

Jerry and I made up, talked it over and went back into counseling.

At times, I felt suffocated. Other times, I felt hopeful. But, most of the time, I felt troubled by his outbursts of anger. I was determined to *change him*. We continued in therapy for another couple of years. "What's wrong with me?" I asked my therapist. "The only problem with you" she said to me once, "is that you believe that you are doing something wrong. Deep inside, you feel as though you deserve to be punished." Her message really impacted me. Of course, it made perfect sense. My whole life, since I was born, had been a series of punishments and accusations. If others were not punishing me, I punished myself. Like Jerry, I had to work on my own self-esteem, big time!

The work seemed to be paying off as we looked deeper into our mutual unhealed pasts. Layers of insecurities were slowly being peeled off as well as the lack of trust, anger, jealousy, resentment, and fear.

Not everything was wrong in our relationship. In spite of our challenges and difficulties, we also experienced tremendous moments of joy, adventures, fun, travel, and surprises.

Expanding our horizons together, we worked as a team. I was the dreamer, and while I created the vision board in my mind, Jerry was a willing participant. That's how buying our dream home became a reality in 1992. That house was so grand and beautiful beyond our wildest dreams. We often hosted parties with friends and had many family gatherings. It was a fantastic time! Together, we were exploring life as we never had the chance to do before.

On our birthdays, we would surprise each other with unexpected trips. One day I told Jerry "Pack your suitcase, I'm taking you somewhere. Bring a suit, a bathing suit, shorts, t-shirts, and a passport. We're leaving next week." He was so excited! Like a little kid, he obediently packed his suitcase. He found out where we were headed only when we arrived at the gate and saw the flight departing for Mexico for a very romantic weekend.

Another time, he was surprised to be landing in San Diego, with a convertible waiting for us at the airport, to go to the Ritz Carlton in Laguna Miguel. He loved those surprises so much that he did the same for me— taking me for a spa week in Sonoma, Napa Valley, and a trip to San Francisco.

Both being romantics, we loved to listen to our favorite songs. One night, we fell asleep while floating on an inflated boat in our pool in the backyard. We spent many hours in front of the fireplace in our bedroom, looking at the flames, drinking wine, and sharing memories of the past while trying to build new ones. Every Saturday, without fail, Jerry bought me a bouquet of beautiful flowers consisting of all kinds and of every color. On special occasions and sometimes for no reason at all, roses were delivered to my office with a note saying: "Just because...I love you so."

During football season, we drove to Tucson every weekend to watch the University of Arizona college football games. The main purpose was to see Tiamo, who was attending that college at the time. We would rent a room at a nearby hotel and Tiamo would stay with us for the weekend. Before driving Tiamo back to campus, we would have breakfast together, laugh about stupid things, and talk about serious things too. Jerry loved Tiamo as his own son. Jerry's kids often came to visit us and we had a blast with them too. I dearly loved them and felt close to them as well.

Even Jerry's mother would often come to visit us. Despite the difficulties Jerry experienced with his mom, I found her to be a very fun woman. She loved to laugh and lived life to the fullest. One of her favorite things to do was to go gambling, a favorite that eventually became an addiction for Jerry. They both loved to escape to the world of slot machines.

Circumstances often brought me back to Canada. To the exception of visiting Ross, who lived in Montreal, I went back for funerals or to visit sick family members. So many difficult memories flooded my mind each time I landed on the grounds of my childhood. Some of them I wished I could forget forever.

My father died the year we moved into our dream home. I went to visit him when he was in the hospital. He was diagnosed with terminal cancer and Alzheimer's. He was still in good enough condition to see visitors and I wanted to see him. My father loved music. I gathered his favorites and brought him his cassette player. He looked very happy to see me. My father was not a talker, and after a few words were exchanged, we sat on his hospital bed and listened to the music together. He loved it and smiled. Happy memories seemed to come to his mind. He was so happy, that he ate the entire box of chocolates that I had given him.

When the time came for his dinner and with permission from his doctor, I took him out to eat. In spite of my giving him plenty of choices from the nearby restaurants, his preference was a hamburger, French fries, and a coke. We ate in silence without any eye contact. I reflected back and recalled how he was never really able to look me straight in the eye. What was it that he didn't want to see?

Many times in my life, I've noticed that I would hear a word, read a sentence, or hear a song playing in just the perfect moment. I've learned to pay attention to that. So that night, I called a cab to take my father and I back to the hospital. We both sat in the back seat. Dad was looking out the window, already absent. Silence always had made my father uncomfortable. "Can you put some music on?" he asked the cab driver. I'll never forget what I heard next. It was a song by Barbara Streisand called *Papa, Can You Hear Me* from the movie *Yentl.* Just recently, when I was writing the first part of this book, that song came back to memory and I cried. I loved my father, regardless.

When we arrived in his hospital room, after making sure he changed into pajamas, the time came to say goodbye. I hugged him and told him "I love you, papa." He said "Me too France, I always did." When I left and turned around, I saw him standing at the doorstep of his hospital room. He was still there watching me leave. He looked so small and frail in his lined navy blue and white pajamas. That was the last time I saw him.

My dad was the funniest man alive. He was sharp and witty. That's what people appreciated the most about him. He loved to laugh and found enjoyment in the laughter of other people. He was a wonderful chef and was a self-taught "Homme a tout faire" and a very hard worker. He adored my mother. She was the love of his life.

Three years following the death of my father, my mother died of a stroke. The three of us, Regine, Yvanne, and I went to see her while she was hospitalized. Although she seemed to be recovering and doing well, she died of complications one month later. It was very difficult for me to lose my mom. I always felt very close to her. Even if I had a hard time understanding the reasons behind her lack of protection against my father, I had many more reasons to admire her for her intelligence, determination, wisdom, discretion, kindness, her avant-garde. And in many ways, she was more advanced than her era permitted. She had an open mind and was a survivor.

Sometimes, I hear her laughter in my mind, which brings me to tears. I wish she could have laughed more. There was always such sadness in her eyes, so many unspoken words, and so much kept inside. In spite of everything, I knew that she had loved us very much. And as I look at the portrait of her hanging on my wall, I hear the poem that she used to recite when my parents had guests over, "O Mere, je vous aime tant" which means, "Oh Mother, I love you so." Thank you, Mom, for the privilege of being your daughter.

In addition to everything else that was happening, my oldest sister Regine was then diagnosed with stage 3 breast cancer. I visited her in Montreal on her birthday. She was not doing well. She still suffered horrible migraines and was very thin. She had lost her hair because of the chemotherapy. That really was the most difficult stage of her life. But, she survived the cancer, and is still in remission after eighteen years.

Regine was born prematurely. She had a twin sister, Danielle, who died after eighteen hours with a heart problem. Regine weighed only two pounds and struggled to survive. From the moment of her birth, she was hooked to tubes in an incubator and was fed intravenously. At the age of six, while crossing the street, she was run over by a drunk driver. Half of her scalp had been ripped off. After many plastic surgeries, the doctors gave her a new forehead from the skin taken from her thigh. Possibly due to that accident, she suffered very debilitating migraines throughout her life.

While Regine was dealing with her health issues, so was Yvanne. She developed asthma and allergies that eventually turned into migraine headaches. She, like my oldest sister, was prescribed the same drug called Imitrex. She was still fighting bouts of depression and was seeing a therapist. But, she was still sober. We often saw each other and would have nights out that consisted of long talks over dinner, usually followed by a little shopping. She tried to remain positive, but was struggling. She often felt lonely and wanted to be involved in a serious romantic relationship, which never seemed to work out because she was always getting involved with the *wrong guy*.

THEN CAME 1999, A YEAR I WILL NEVER FORGET

It was Saturday evening and Jerry and I had just settled down in the family room to watch a movie after dinner. The phone rang. Not having my handset with me, I went into the den to answer the call.

"Hello, are you France Barringer?" asked a male voice on the phone. "Yes, I am" I replied, perplexed as I saw the police identification on the caller ID. "This is Officer Robert from the Phoenix Police Department, ma'am. I don't have good news to tell you and I want to make sure that you are not alone right now." "No, I am not alone" I said. "My husband is with me. Please, tell me what this is about." "It's about your sister, Yvanne" he continued. "She has been found dead in her apartment. It is obvious that it is a suicide, as she left you a letter to that effect. My partner and I will take that letter to you right now along with some of her personal belongings. Please give us your address and we will leave immediately."

Still holding the phone in one hand and trying to understand what was happening, I pulled out a chair from under the desk and sat down. I gave the officer our address and hung up. It was semi-dark in the den. I could only see the light from the living room window across the room. By staring at the lights, it was as though I was taken away from the words I had just heard. My little sister was dead!

"Honey what's going on?" Jerry asked. I got up, picked up the phone again, and hoped that maybe the officer would call back and say "We are so sorry, we made a terrible mistake. She is still alive." Then, I could go and see her in the hospital, like I had done before, and I would hold her once more.

I walked back into the family room and saw my husband sitting on the leather couch in front of the television set. "What's going on?" he asked again. I was afraid to give life to the words. I sat down and blurted out "Yvanne killed herself. The police are coming over." At that moment, I noticed my pink long night gown was soaking wet. I was drenched in perspiration. "Oh my God Honey!" he said, trying to hold me in his arms. For some reason, I couldn't be held and I felt like I couldn't breathe. My head was spinning, and my heart was beating so hard in my chest. I sat there and gave Jerry my hand to hold. I became conscious of my body again and noticed a sharp pain in my throat. I couldn't cry, and I was so cold! Trembling, I grabbed the white and green throw from the couch and wrapped it around myself.

"Let's have a glass of wine while waiting for the police" Jerry said. Like a robot, I followed him into the kitchen and sat down with him at the table. I drank the whole glass in one sip.

A few minutes later, the officer and his female partner arrived. Jerry led them both in the kitchen where the four of us sat. The officer opened up a brown envelope that contained a letter addressed to me, part in French, part in English. He then opened a bag and pulled out articles that were found on Yvanne's kitchen table. Inside the bag was a book opened up to a specific page, a bible opened up to a specific highlighted verse, her pink pajamas that I had given her, and the watch that she was wearing when she was found. It was the watch I had given her…the day she admired it on me. The last item he pulled out of the bag was a long pendant with an attached crucifix. The officer was speaking words I didn't hear. I was only able to look at the objects he was displaying on the table. There was another letter, which gave instructions on how to contact me.

Yvanne thought of everything! Every detail was carefully planned, even the objects that I was staring at on the table. I heard the officer's voice again. He was reading details from the police report about how she was found—sitting on a chair facing the kitchen table, in her pink pajamas, a mask covered her mouth, her head tilted to the right, enveloped in a plastic bag that was secured with a rubber band around her neck. The suicidal instruction book she had underlined the suicide process from, was opened in front of her. On the table was the letter addressed to me and the bible. She was wearing a crucifix and my watch. She barricaded herself inside her apartment and the police had to break in through the balcony.

"My poor little sister" I thought. "What have you done?!"

Then, the female officer specializing in suicide cases gave me instructions on how to get help. She left pamphlets on the table. "Any questions?" she asked. "None" I replied. All questions had been answered. The evidence was all there, along with what was left of her. I called my sister Regine in Montreal, and my son Tiamo in Virginia. Ross and I were in non-speaking terms since my birthday, the previous year.

I couldn't sleep that night. I looked at the watch I had given her and it was no longer working. The same thing happened with my father's watch. Even though I had it repaired, it never worked after he passed away. I put Yvanne's watch around my wrist, and then I lay down on the couch and exploded in sobs. *A part of me was gone.*

I spoke to Yvanne the day of her death. I called her at lunchtime, eager to share that I had found a solution to her problems. She was so depressed and her medication was not working. I wanted her to be hospitalized and under supervision. I thought that surely the doctors could find a medication that could work for her. I told Yvanne my idea and offered to pay for her hospital care. Yvanne said "I'll think about it France and I'll let you know when I call you on Sunday." Then, she called back at 3:00 pm that same day and said "I love you very much, France." Those are the last words I heard from her.

After her call, I couldn't help but feel an extreme sadness in me. Driving home from work that day, I felt an overwhelming wave of pain wash over me as if I was hit by a tsunami. I drove home crying the whole way and not understanding why. It's as though I heard her voice in my head that said "I'm sorry." Yvanne was fifty-two years old.

I had a dream a month before her death. We were both walking on the side of a cliff. The cliff was grey, and it was grey outside. In the dream, Yvanne told me that she wanted to jump, as she looked down at the bottom of the cliff. I held her hand, she looked at me, and then she let go of my hand and jumped off into nothingness. I shared that dream with her. She cried.

Two years before her suicide, she was hospitalized for the third time. She had taken a bunch of pills. Her friend received a letter from her and called 911. I also received a letter, but I was out of town. When I returned home, I found out that she was in the hospital. Fifteen years of therapy had done nothing to help her. She never recovered from my father's beatings and was constantly seeking to be loved by him, through relationships that never worked out. Each suicide attempt came after a break up. She overcame everything else in her life, except that.

The Three Funerals

I held a service for Yvanne in Phoenix a few days following her suicide. A lot of people came to say goodbye, perhaps as many as sixty people. Beautiful flowers were delivered, including one gorgeous bouquet of white and red roses in the shape of a heart from her very close friends that loved her so much. Many people came to speak of her—her elegance, her charm, and her smile. They spoke about her funny ways, her generosity, and the compassion she felt for others. They shared about the support she gave others, in spite of her needing so much, and how she asked so little of others. People emphasized her sense of humor, charisma, and the love she showed clients while making them feel beautiful by styling their hair and listening to their problems. Many people at the service were crying, but they were also laughing and remembering the silly things she had done. Yet, very few people knew of her pain, with the exception of her best friend Pauline, her sponsor Maggie, and her therapist. The few that knew, did not let anyone know about Yvanne's depression and her suicide. The instructions that Yvanne left me were very clear; "Say that I died of an asthma attack" she wrote in her letter. So, that's what I did. I don't think people believed me, but what did it matter? She was gone!

Two days later, I left for Canada. I carried her ashes in my carry-on luggage. From the start, it was a trip from hell. One hour into the flight to Toronto, we turned around because of a mechanical malfunction, as it was losing power. After waiting many hours in the airport for the problem to be fixed, I missed my connection in Toronto and I arrived very late that night in Montreal. The airline lost my luggage, but it was later found and delivered to me two days later. Yvanne's second funeral was held in Roxboro, outside Montreal. It was for my father's side of the family. I saw the aunt that took care of me when I was four years old. Yvanne's favorite aunt and godmother were also there. Ross came to give his support and we were speaking again. The following day, I left for Disraeli, the town where my parents lived and were buried. My sister, Regine and my brother-in-law, Mike were with me.

When we arrived at the church for the service held for my mother's side of the family, I felt exhausted! It was the last destination. In church, I looked at Yvanne's picture on display in front of the urn and I remembered when it was taken. We went out shopping together one evening and she tried on a beautiful purple outfit. When she came out of the dressing room and saw how stunning she looked, I took her picture to capture her beautiful smile. We both laughed and went to dinner.

This last funeral was by far the most difficult. A few steps away from the church was the cemetery. It was cold and rainy outside. That's how I felt inside. When the service was over, I walked toward the cemetery with the urn in my arms. Regine walked besides me and asked, "France, can I hold her too?" I thought "I held her all my life alone and I will continue to do so until the end." Then, I realized Regine was suffering too. As I gave her the urn, she said "No, let's carry her together." So, we both carried the urn until we arrived at the designated hole in the ground. We put her in the bottom of the hole and said our final good bye. On the headstone it was written: "My sister, with the most beautiful smile in the world 1947 - 1999." I looked up in front of me and there was a beautiful view of the lake. Regine and I held each other. Mike came and covered us with an umbrella. It was time to leave her, to leave them—my mom, my dad, and my beloved sister, Yvanne.

Slowly, we walked towards the car, not looking back. Regine and I were huddled under the same umbrella, with her hand covering mine. I sat in the backseat. I was so cold. I looked out the window and thought to myself, *another cycle has ended.* Mike turned on the radio and incredibly, "Alors Adieu" was playing by Alain Barriere.

And, a new cycle began.

In June of 2000, Jerry and I put our dream home on the market for sale. We were downsizing to a smaller home, in preparation for Jerry's retirement in six years. Tiamo, after living in Virginia for two years, was coming back home. After his graduation from college, in May of 1998, Tiamo announced to me one day, that he desired to venture into unknown territory and move to Virginia. A sense of adventure and exploration was brewing inside of him. He packed all that he could take with him and bought a one-way ticket for the Greyhound bus heading for Virginia. Later, he wrote a song about that three-day trip titled "From AZ to VA."

Jerry flew to Virginia, rented a truck, and helped Tiamo move across country. It took them three days to drive back. This time, it was from VA to AZ. In the meantime, we received an excellent offer on our home. It was a smart decision to downsize, but I felt extremely sad to sell the home we had lived in for 8 years. That house had a soul. A soul that Jerry, Tiamo, and I formed together.

So many memories filled my mind as I sat on the living room steps on our moving day. My eyes welled up with tears when I thought back to 1992—when the three of us drove up to the house one day to celebrate because the foundation had been poured in. We brought candles, a portable cassette player and stopped at Burger King on the way.

As we sat there eating our burgers, we recalled what led us to choose this house on the final home-selection weekend. Tiamo was very much involved in the decision-making process and was thirteen years old at the time. Jerry and I had our top three homes for him to choose from. Uncertain about the possibilities and afraid of being disappointed, Tiamo asked me "Are any of these dream homes even possible to dream about, Mom?" "We don't know yet Tiamo" I said. "But once we make a selection, we'll find out." Then he asked "But why am I dreaming of things that may not even happen?" "Because, to make them happen, you have to dream of them first" I replied, holding his hand.

And on that selection-weekend, the last home we saw was the one that spoke to our collective hearts. As Tiamo walked below the archway between the kitchen and living room area, he exclaimed "This is the one!" And then he added "It feels so right, right here, right now." Jerry and I looked at each other and united, we concluded; "This is the one then. It's decided!"

A year later, as we looked at that same archway, we smiled as we lit candles while the sun was setting. It was a very solemn moment. Now living in our dream home, the three of us recalled that instant in time where the dream was created. Inspired by the soft candlelight, we transported ourselves into beautiful, magical lands while listening to the soundtrack music from the movie "Somewhere in Time." We had imagined, constructed, built, and manifested a dream that was now real in *concrete,* on solid ground. In that ceremony, we added a soul to the home.

It was a combination of love, hope, joy and unity—*a trinity…Somewhere in Time.*

Eight years later, it was as though Tiamo had come back to say good-bye to the home we so loved. We sold the house the same month that he moved back to Arizona. Moving day was one of the saddest days of my life. I argued with myself and thought "It's just a house, France. Why such sadness?" That's just it! It was not just a house. It was an unforgettable period in time that I didn't want to leave behind. It was a miracle, because we believed. Just like a *gift from Santa Claus.*

As fate would have it, our moving day was October 19, 2000—the one-year anniversary day of Yvanne's death.

As we downsized to a smaller home, the company I was working for was downsizing too. I lost my job the day after we closed escrow. Coincidence or destiny? I was fifty-two years old.

And with one more move into a new home, a new cycle began again.

During the next five years after losing my job, I ventured into new careers other than the world of technology that I was trained in. According to the industry, I was getting *too old* for the market. So I became a fashion consultant and had my own business for a while. I then worked in the designer department for Saks Fifth Avenue. And then in 2002, I became a realtor. That same year, Tiamo moved to San Diego. During that period of time, I often felt sorry for myself. I drank alone in the evening to soothe the anxiety that I was increasingly feeling. It became a vicious cycle. I drank to forget that I was depressed and then became more depressed because I was drinking too much.

One day, on July 15, 2004 I made a life-changing decision. "I am done!" I declared to my dear friend Pauline. I gave her my insurance information and asked her to make arrangements for me to go to a detoxification center. I also asked her to pick me up as soon as my treatment would be completed. When I requested that of her, I knew that I would keep my word. I didn't want to fail. Pauline drove me to the center and stayed with me for five hours, which was the time it took for a bed to become available, because someone had to be discharged first. I saw people coming in and out. Some left and ran off for one last drink. Each time I went to the bathroom while waiting, I looked at a painting that hung from a wall in the hallway. It was a very simple painting of a road, nothing else, but the words above the road said *Believe that you can.* I believed, and I knew that I could. In fact, I was walking on that road. I haven't touched a drink since that day.

The following year, we sold the house and after a few months of renting, made the decision to buy another house. Unfortunately, with the real estate market being so high, we had to move further away to the southeast outskirts of Phoenix to a suburb called Queen Creek. It was very far away and we were isolated from everyone. Jerry retired in 2006, the same year we bought the new house in Queen Creek.

Another move, another cycle.

I felt very alone in Queen Creek. I was no longer working. I submerged myself in books, online classes, and workshops all on spiritual growth. Then over the next few years, I was frequently having heart palpitations. Sometimes, I felt very dizzy to the point of almost fainting. On more rare occasions, I even felt as though my heart was stopping. The cardiologist couldn't find anything wrong.

After retiring, Jerry became very bored and we were not getting along. Our relationship was deteriorating. We argued most of the time and never seemed to find resolution between us. Unhappy, Jerry was eating and drinking more and I submerged myself even deeper into my own interior life. I felt alone and distressed, which was not what I had envisioned for the rest of my life. But, I was determined to change my situation.

The Day I Left

A few days after my sixtieth birthday, following an argument with Jerry that was no more serious than previous ones, I packed a large suitcase and called Tiamo. "I'm leaving Jerry; can you pick me up at the airport today?" "Sure, Mom, let me know what time and I'll be there." Reassured, I called my friend Pauline to take me to the airport and I booked the next flight to San Diego.

Many difficulties were ahead of me. Our savings were basically depleted with the house we purchased in Queen Creek. I felt so uncertain about the life ahead of me, but couldn't live the life I was currently in either. I found myself at a crossroads again. I was exhausted from the senseless arguments between Jerry and me, and once again, Ross and I were no longer speaking for an extended period of time. We had been in and out of communication so many times, as a result of always trying to mend the past—a past that never healed and kept showing up in the present. I had to start all over again.

I felt that my life was always about starting over. This time, I was sixty years old. There was something to be said about being sixty. I worked my whole life and overcame so much. But instead of resting and enjoying life, I had to do it all over again. How was I going to make it? I didn't have a clue.

A few days later, Jerry realized that I was not coming back. He was writing emails and wanted to communicate. He wanted to understand, he wanted to change. For three weeks we wrote each other. I was still not going back. But then, one day I opened my email to find a letter from him. He had attempted suicide but couldn't go through with it.

He desperately wanted me back and told me he would do anything. "Make a list of what you need from me" he asked. "I will do whatever it takes to have you back."

So I created a list and wanted to believe him. He agreed to immediately go into counseling to deal with his anger issues. We had a plan. After many emails and phone calls, I decided to go back for Christmas. Tiamo was planning to come back with me. In the meantime, Ross and I had re-opened the communication between us as we had spoken on the phone a couple of times.

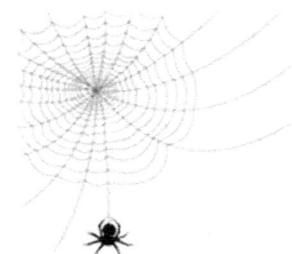

Was it possible to mend all of these broken hearts at once?

As I am writing this and looking outside my window, I see an intricate spider web hanging from a branch in a tree. I am in awe, observing the spider's masterpiece being built. One by one, she forms a thread and takes it all the way to the opposite end. She then returns, walking back on the same thread and constructs another one, going in another direction. Who directs her? How does she know where to go, what to do? How does she know where to go and I do not? She is following a master plan. Am I?

Was it in my master plan to go back home? I didn't know the answer. Like the spider, I was walking back on the same thread to build another one, in another direction. Like her, I would have to find out the results of my efforts, once I was done building my masterpiece. If I were to know the results, would I build it?

The day Tiamo and I were going back to Arizona for Christmas, I received an email from Ross telling me that he didn't want to speak to me ever again. Why was he breaking the thread we were trying to build? So many of them had been broken in the past by either one of us. How very strange! And as I opened the door to return home, another door was closing at the same time.

Going Back

As Tiamo and I were driving back to Arizona, a song by Leigh Nash *Nervous In The Light Of Dawn* was playing. As I listened to the lyrics, with tears in my eyes, I turned my head and looked at Tiamo. We often spoke in silence, beyond what words can say. Holding the wheel with his left hand, he extended his right hand to hold one of mine. For a few minutes, we drove like that, in the awareness of the events that were unfolding in my life. *In that very moment, holding his hand, I felt so safe!*

Six hours later, we arrived. Jerry came outside to greet us. He held me and cried.

That Christmas, Tiamo gave me a unique gift wrapped in three different packages. In one box was a pine cone, in another was a key, and in the last box was an apple pie. Those were the clues given to me to guess what my real gift was. It turned out that my gift was for the two of us to go to a small, cozy town in northern Arizona called Strawberry. When he was a little boy and as a young teenager, I often took him there. It was our special getaway. I would rent a room with a fireplace. We would have dinner in the restaurant seated by the stone fireplace, and then eat their homemade apple pie a la mode. Sometimes we played Yahtzee, a fun board game that we both enjoyed. In the morning, we would have pancakes and then go for a walk in the woods. We hadn't done that in years! So, the two of us took off for Strawberry, two days after Christmas.

I gave Tiamo a dream board on that same Christmas. He started to build his dream of becoming a successful full-time singer/songwriter in place of his day job. Another dream of his was to meet his soul mate. He succeeded in attracting all of his dreams.

Meanwhile, I had to redesign my own dream board.

Jerry and I were trying our best, but we had so many difficulties. I felt trapped in my own spider web. In the months following my return to Arizona, I was having more and more heart palpitations. The cardiologist gave me a heart monitor for forty-five days. Wearing the monitor, not once did I have heart palpitations. Go figure! One day, I was having lunch with my very dear friend, Pauline. All of sudden, my heart started beating so fast and it was out of control. As we decided to go to the emergency room, the palpitations stopped on the way. I decided to go home and rest.

As soon as I got home, the palpitations started again, but this time they wouldn't stop. Jerry drove me to the closest emergency heart hospital, forty-five minutes away from home. By the time we got there, my heart was flopping in my chest, from left to right as if it was Jell-O pudding. My heartbeat indicated 273 beats per minute, and the doctor intravenously induced a solution to lower my heart rate. It only worked for a couple of minutes. The doctor had to jumpstart my heart in order to bring it back to a normal rate. That procedure stabilized me enough until I had surgery two days later.

I had a condition called "supraventricular tachycardia", which has to do with an abnormal fast heart rhythm. A normal heart rate varies between 60 to 100 beats per minute. After the surgery one morning, the nurse transferred to me a telephone call. "Hello" I said, not knowing who was on the line. "Mom, hi it's Ross. How are you?" he asked. It had been three years since we last spoke. As we talked, I was looking at the beautiful green and white bouquet of flowers that had just been delivered from him. "Hi Ross, I'm fine. Thank you so much for the beautiful flowers. I love them. It's a gorgeous bouquet!" I replied. "I am glad you like it" he responded, as if all was normal again. "Mom, if you want to move on, I'm ready to move on. Are you?" he asked. "Yes, I am son, I'm ready to move on" I happily replied.

Did the spider go back into the web and pick up the thread that she had left unfinished?

Or, was she creating a new one?

She decided that it was time for a new thread to be built.

"We are moving to San Diego" I once said to Jerry. Neither Jerry nor I liked Queen Creek. The real estate market had taken a major plunge and we had to let go of the house. Prior to even knowing how we would move to San Diego, or when, we sold all of our furniture and had garage sales every weekend. Then, on June 25, 2010, we took off for San Diego with a moving truck! I had lived in Arizona for thirty-three years.

And, *another cycle had just begun.*

Despite the successful heart surgery, I still had heart-racing palpitations combined with dizziness. After numerous tests, I was told that all was in order. Frustrated, I kept a journal of all the physical symptoms I was experiencing corresponding to the emotions I was feeling. I suspected that subconsciously, I was carrying unhealed emotions from the past. My body was yelling for me to pay attention. To what? I didn't know anymore. I looked and searched for answers numerous times before, how was it going to be any different that time? Keeping a daily log of the symptoms and emotions was just not enough.

Determined to find answers one day, instead of my usual journal writing, I closed my eyes and invited my subconscious mind to be my guide. Fearless, I asked, "What is it that you want me to see? What am I hiding? What am I protecting?" And, as I stepped away from my conscious mind, I started writing—the writing that created this book.

The more I wrote, the more I felt. The more I felt, the more unfolded. Layers upon layers of grief, anguish, and torment were surfacing. Unprotected, the pain had nowhere to hide anymore. Fear was the monster that had attacked me when I was defenseless at two years of age. For all of my life, my countless efforts in trying to escape the fear were useless. It followed me everywhere I went—even in my dreams. In the middle of the night, there were many times when I abruptly woke myself up by screaming the most dreadful and terrifying screams.

There was nowhere to run to anymore. Instead, *I just stood still*. I invited fear and its many forms to speak to me. I closed my eyes and asked "Please show yourself to me." And then it appeared, like a shadow, in front of me. I looked at it straight on and asked "What is your purpose in my life?" Fear's answer came unexpectedly, "I served my purpose, now that you are willing to look at me." Like a child who just woke up from a nightmare, I was becoming more and more aware and awakened. I realized that the nightmare was over.

As I continued purging all of my deepest emotions, so was my body. For six months, I had bouts of diarrhea and had to run to the bathroom twelve to fifteen times a day. I lost fifteen pounds in the process.

Like a snake shedding its old skin, I was shedding my old ways. A new me was emerging. All of my life, I fought battles. I was done fighting. "Give it all up!" I wrote one day. Give up changing Jerry, my children, my friends, or anyone or anything outside of me. The only one I could really change and transform was *me*. While I was losing weight, Jerry was gaining it. His health was suffering greatly. He was forced to make a change. So many of us suffer before we make better choices. Yet, life becomes so beautiful when we choose to listen to our higher knowing. We always get another chance. But, that chance is always up to us to take or leave.

Jerry chose to take that chance and started his own healing journey into self-discovery. He lost over one hundred pounds, walking an average of fifteen miles a day. Walking that many miles, day after day, opened his heart. His journey was being defined in front of his eyes. He became a walking meditation, communing with the Divine within. While he was shedding the pounds, his anger was leaving him and self-love was replacing it. He is now a transformed man!

In my process of letting go, I realized there was still more to let go of. Three of my friends died last year. One of them was a shaman that I dearly loved. It was hard to slowly see him leave. He died on June 5, 2012, when Venus transitioned between the earth and the sun, a rare alignment that occurred over a century ago. The night he died, was when I arrived in Canada to visit my son, Ross. Planets transit, and so do humans. I said goodbye to my friend, as I said hello to my son.

OUR LIVES ARE ENDLESS CIRCLES, FILLED WITH ENDINGS AND BEGINNINGS.

THE END, *OR IS IT JUST THE BEGINNING?*

As I contemplated about these cycles, unexpectedly, one day I looked up in the mirror, and there she was! A wise, little two year old girl. She looked into my eyes and said to me...

"You have done well. You have returned to where it all started.

When you embarked on this journey you call your life, I was here all along with you.

Together, we fought battles and together, we are coming home.

I have learned so much from you and I promise I will never forget it.

I will remind you always that:

I am at all times here speaking to you. Just listen.

If you can't hear me, I will speak louder until you can hear me.

Each time you sit by a tree, you are never alone.

Each time you build a dream, there is a Santa Claus.

Each time you help someone, you wipe your own tears.

Each time you forgive, you heal your own wounds.

Each time you fail and dare to try again, you succeed.

Each time you stop judging yourself, you accept someone else.

Each time you listen to someone's life story, you are writing your own.

Each time you doubt, you learn about faith.

Each time you hope, you create an opportunity.

Each time there is an ending, there is a new beginning.

Each time you hear a beautiful symphony, you are a note being played.

Each time you look at the ocean, you are a wave.

Each time you look up at the stars, a light appears in your eyes.

That light that I see in your eyes, is called love.

A love that is eternal, that never left you, and never will.

And, *each time you feel broken*, I will remind you that you have been made whole a long time ago and you only forgot."

"Rebecca, are you asleep?" asked the lady, looking at her little squirrel friend lying by her side. "Oh no" replied Rebecca. "I heard every single word. And now that I know what love is, I can go home and tell Johnny." "What will you tell him?" Rebecca curiously asked. "I will tell him that love is not something you ask for, or hear from another, but that love is something *you are* and must recognize in yourself, to see it in another. I will tell him to look deep into my eyes to see my very soul. And when I will look into his eyes, *I will see him for the very first time*" Rebecca concluded.

The end, *or is it just the beginning?*

This is what my new beginning is, in this moment as I am writing these words. My marriage is continuously transforming into the peacefulness I always yearned for. My relationship with my oldest son Ross is filled with love, mutual forgiveness, tenderness, and a greater appreciation of our relationship. Rather than focusing on the fight for survival and falling victim to my life challenges, I now filter my energy and time into my new life purpose. Today, I feel vibrant and alive, as I have shed a lifetime of painful experiences, and have stepped into the love of who I truly am.

Now, I want to show you the path that I took to get me where I am today—where it is safe, and that you are loved for exactly who you are. This you will find, as I walk with you through the journey of my healing. This next chapter is your chapter—your chapter in overcoming your deepest hurts, and finding a new opening to your spirit that has been waiting for you to discover.

And, that will be your own new beginning. Go forth now. Your spirit is waiting.

From left to right, Yvanne Regine and me

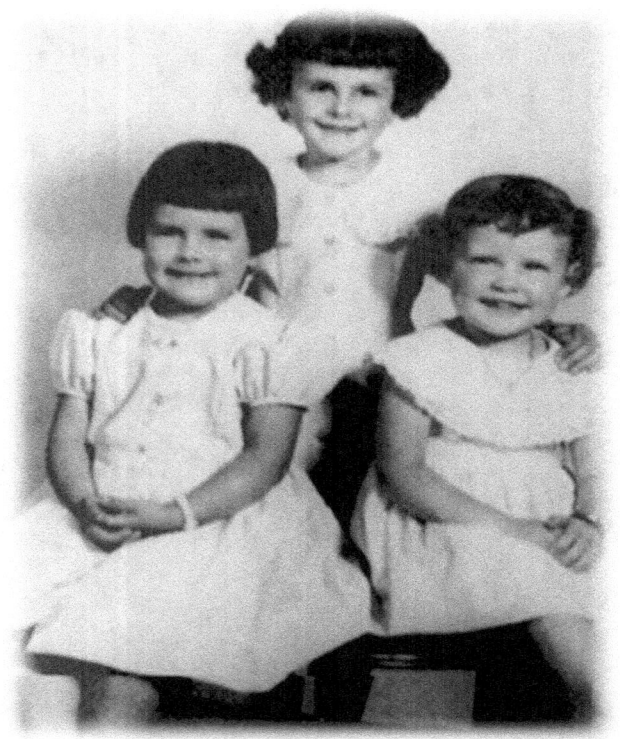

END